What Was I Thinking?
Toxic Shock Syndrome (TSS)

by

Dr. Patrick M Schlievert

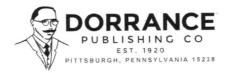

DORRANCE
PUBLISHING CO
EST. 1920
PITTSBURGH, PENNSYLVANIA 15238

Dorrance Publishing Co
585 Alpha Drive
Pittsburgh, PA 15238
Visit our website at *www.dorrancebookstore.com*

ISBN: 978-1-6480-4246-1
eISBN: 978-1-6480-4685-8

Dedication

This book is dedicated my wife Shirley and my daughter Sara
for their continued love and support over the many years this book
was in the making.

What Was I Thinking?
Toxic Shock Syndrome (TSS)

by

Dr. Patrick M Schlievert

"All the world's a stage,
And all the men and women merely players;
They have their exits and their entrances;
And one man in his time plays many parts…"

From: *As You Like It*
Spoken by: Jaques
Written by: William Shakespeare

"All the World's a stage
And men, and only a few women
Are thinking about their lines in this play,
While most are not…"

Written by: Patrick M. Schlievert

Chapter 1

What I Was Thinking?

I have been on a long, winding adventure, beginning in the summer of 1978 and continuing even up to the spring of 2020, pursuing important, serious diseases that reportedly did not exist but in fact did exist, ultimately resulting in extensive and critical broad-spectrum mass media news coverage. I hope to take you on an expedition with me through this disease and additionally, into the depths of science in hopefully an easy way to understand but more importantly, to lead you through the complex web of pure speculation, pseudoscience, and real science that gave rise to our understanding and misunderstanding of these new diseases called toxic shock syndromes (hereon known by the initials TSS). TSS is a one of-a-kind infection caused by two kinds of bacteria, where speculation, pseudoscience, and real science are impressively and openly on display for you to see, real time as they unfolded, many times spectacularly. Please read on, and I think you will see that TSS has as much pure speculation and pseudoscience, in the name of reality, as it has real science. Perhaps surprisingly, despite the significant problems, I think we have a pretty good understanding of the clinical disease, though not the full spectrum, many but not all epidemiological risk factors, and parts of the microbiology and immunology underpinning the unique causes. At the same time, we still have so much to learn.

Overall, I sometimes feel like I am moving a sludge pile forward, because when I push important new disease aspects forward, irrelevant things oftentimes ooze out the side, become important for only a brief period of time, get in the way of important scientific advances but ultimately are thrown into the trash heap where they belong. The TSS field then again moves forward.

It would be helpful if the biomedical science community for one just one time could see TSS as important. This disease is the major reason more than one hundred thousand Americans die of *Staphylococcus aureus* and *Streptococcus pyogenes* infections, directly or secondarily to other diseases, each year. I am adding here a list of four scientific references that will address in detail the number of cases of the various staphylococcal and streptococcal diseases in the United States each year.[1,2,3,4] Since this book is written primarily for the American public, I do not want to burden you unnecessarily with references. I will place some very important ones at appropriate places, and you can find them listed at the end of the book.

I am reminded of what a famous university microbiology professor communicated to me several years ago: "Pat, now that you have described the toxin that causes TSS and there is nothing left to discover, what are you going to do with the rest of your life?" What was he thinking?

My immediate response to him was: "I think I will find a few new things to do... like new things for the rest of my career, unraveling two of the most interesting diseases that reportedly did not exist, but did in fact exist." I hope this book tells you what I, and others, have done that is important for biomedical science but mostly for your well being.

As you read this book, consider the following question, as in the book title: "What was I (Patrick Schlievert) thinking?" However, in many examples with bad advice and bad patient outcomes, perhaps you should be asking: "What were THEY thinking?" That is for sure what I was thinking at the time.

I have a few disclaimers before I get too far into this book. First, I was labeled, by my high school graduating classmates, most likely to become a nuclear physicist. This was the nerdiest thing they could come up with for me. I am sure they would have found something more nerdy to say if there was such a thing. They may even have tattooed on my chest: "NERD". I wear it as a badge of honor though. While I did not become a nuclear physicist, I did become a scientist, and

2

I did become an amateur astrophysicist, including making a spectroscope back in eighth grade to look at the stars. From *Dictionary.com* a spectroscope is "an optical device for producing and observing a spectrum of light or radiation from any source, consisting essentially of a slit through which the radiation passes, a collimating lens, and an Amici prism." What the hell did I just say?

Second, I am a lot older than Dr. Neil deGrasse Tyson, Astrophysicist and Frederick P. Rose, Director of the Hayden Planetarium at the Rose Center for Earth and Space in New York City. However, in this book I try to adhere to factual thinking, like him, and present findings and discussions as real as possible. Neil deGrasse Tyson has made it well known that he dislikes it when movies, books, and particularly scientists, do things or make alien beings that do not follow the universal laws of physics. I will follow the universal laws of microbiology and immunology.

I have been thinking recently, which can be a dangerous thing to do these days. I think I can define time as an entity, in other words as a packet that we call "time". Time cannot, for example, be infinitely small or infinitely large. Infinitely small means that time can never have any dimensions, such as length, width, height, weight, and temperature. Anything multiplied by infinitely small remains infinitely small. Yet, we know time exists as it passes, and indeed as we age, time seems to go faster and faster. And, then we are gone. Here is what I think is the smallest unit of time: the time it takes a photon of light to travel Planck's length. Planck's length is 1.6×10^{-35} meters; this is the smallest distance named so far. Light travels at 3×10^8 meters per second. Thus, the smallest unit of time must be 5.3×10^{-42} seconds, in which a photon travels Planck's length. In other words, this is a really small but very real number; 5.3 with forty-one zeros and a decimal point in front of it. I think this confirms that I am indeed the nerd my high school graduating class thought I was.

Third, all the things presented in this book are true as they relate to me, and as I remember them. I have a pretty good memory for things. I have named many participating scientists because they merit important recognition for the immense good that they have done to move the TSS research field forward. I name only a few of those who have stood in the way of progress. For many folks who stood in the way, I leave them nameless, so I do not give them credit where credit is not due. Over time, I have come to be what I call "appropriately cynical", possibly because of my upbringing but mostly I think because of living my forty-five years as a research scientist at a university. In this book, I will give you many examples of "appropriate cynicism". I leave it to you to decide if my cynicism is appropriate.

The final disclaimer: You will read that I have PhD and not an MD. Thus, I am not a "real doctor" and cannot practice medicine. I in fact do not practice medicine. So, how can I write this book as if I have an MD degree? A few reasons come to mind. First, I have run over eighteen thousand miles with Dr. Robert Coates, MD, a clinician and dear friend, and we have had endless hours to discuss clinical medicine and clinical cases of all sorts. Second, I have consulted on over eight thousand cases of staphylococcal TSS and more than two thousand cases of streptococcal toxic shock syndrome. This means many physicians ask me for my advice. I may have seen more actual patients with TSS than anyone else, even though I did not participate in their direct disease management and therapy. Many physicians ask my advice, both originating from reading the published scientific literature, where I have over four hundred publications on TSS, and being directed to me from the Centers for Disease Control, and now including Prevention (CDC). I give advice freely and have never charged for this advice. I do qualify my advice, wherein I say to physicians that I will give you my best advice on treatment, but then it is your job to decide how to treat the patient since I am not a physician.

Let me give you examples of how this works. A physician from New York City called me one day on advice given to him from the CDC. This physician had a male, fourteen-year-old patient with hemorrhagic (meaning profuse blood leaking into the lungs) pneumonia and toxic shock syndrome following influenza. The physician was at a complete loss for how to treat the patient, painfully lamenting: "Pat, unless you tell me what to do for treatment, this boy will die tonight. I have done all that I know how to do. I am serious, he will die tonight. The CDC thought you could help me." I first reminded him that I am not a physician. He said that made no difference to him: "Just tell me what to do." I said to give the boy the antibiotic vancomycin to cover for methicillin-resistant *Staphylococcus aureus* (MRSA), the antibiotic clindamycin because it can turn off toxin (poison) production by *Staphylococcus aureus*, even if it cannot kill the microbe, the antibiotic rifampin because of its great penetrating ability into tissues, like the lungs with fluid build-up, and intravenous immunoglobulin. It turns out the boy had hemorrhagic pneumonia and TSS due to MRSA. Thus, vancomycin was critical to kill the MRSA. In addition, TSS is a disease caused by a toxin (poison), so clindamycin may help by preventing the MRSA from secreting its potent toxin into the lungs. Rifampin can penetrate the tissues and fluid well, and although it would never be given alone to treat *Staphylococcus aureus* infections, it synergizes with the other two antibiotics to increase effectiveness. Most importantly, I said to give commercially-available intravenous immunoglobulin since this is a pool of antibodies from thousands of healthy people, and many (80 percent), even if not all people, will have antibodies that can protect the boy from the toxins (poisons) produced by the causative bacteria. The toxins are the things that actually kill the boy. They are not alive, so antibiotics do not affect them. The physician hung up and gave this entire regimen to the boy. The physician called me the next day, a bit overwhelmed but ecstatic. He said: "The boy is so well, he is hopping on his bed, and is well on the way to recovery. No high fever, no shock, and the lungs on the way to clearing." What a great feeling! Think about it... what a great feeling to have had such an impact.

However, I was also called that same prior day by a physician treating a fourteen-year-old girl, the same age as the boy. I was asked to help by the State Health Department (not New York), but the physician chose not to give the treatment I had suggested. After a lot of back-and-forth, including the Health Department asking that I re-give the full-court press one more time, the physician again said no to the use of my suggested treatment. The major problem was, as the physician said: "The intravenous immunoglobulin is expensive and not proven by a case-control study to be effective. Insurance also may not cover its use."

I replied: "Then ask the parents to pay for the intravenous immunoglobulin. Any parent would rather have their daughter alive than dead." I commonly make the following statement as I teach medical students in training to be physicians: "It is better to be alive than dead." The fourteen-year-old daughter died that night. By my reckoning, not using intravenous immunoglobulin was done primarily to save money, as intravenous immunoglobulin at that time was $30,000 per treatment. What were they thinking?

Many physicians ask me to help families cope with daughters who have recovered, or are on the way to recovering, from TSS. Why would physicians ask me to do this? Menstrual toxic shock syndrome is very different from all other diseases. Recurrences happen and are common; up to 40 percent of patients will have recurrences.[5] In other words, immunity to the causative toxin (poison) and bacteria never develops, and patients can have the disease multiple times. I will explain the underlying molecular reason in a later chapter. However, I know of many young women who have been admitted to intensive care units in hospitals up to six times due to recurrences of serious TSS. Some young women have even asked me: "If I have a hysterectomy, will this stop the disease from recurring?" I suggest such treatment is way too radical and unnecessary. They should ask their treating physician for the immunoglobulin treatment mentioned above. This has worked for many patients to prevent recurrences because once the toxin is neutralized, immunity to the bacteria can develop. It turns out that one treatment will do the job. Intravenous immunoglobulin currently now costs about $8000 per treatment.

Some consulting infectious diseases physicians are friends of mine, and at times, they have had trouble convincing primary treating physicians that the patient in fact has menstrual TSS. Menstrual TSS can mimic a variety of other diseases, including autoimmune diseases, where the patient's own immune system is trying to kill her. Unlike autoimmunity where we usually do not know the cause, if you get rid of the causative bacteria in TSS, the autoimmune-appearing TSS goes away. I will give some other examples throughout this book. An aside: wouldn't it be interesting if autoimmune diseases in general were in fact all caused by microorganisms, where we could then treat them with antibiotics instead of just managing symptoms as we currently mostly do? Just watch television and you will see the impressive numbers of expensive agents to manage symptoms of autoimmunity. These agents, almost always monoclonal antibodies, are given over and over again, and this of course feeds into the impressive profits of pharmaceutical companies. It is difficult today to convince United States companies even to develop and produce antibiotics. By their estimation, the profits are simply not high enough. Antibiotics treat the one-time infection and are not needed continuously, as opposed to antibodies that we see advertised all the time on television.

There are what are called delayed sequelae—that is, things that happen to the patient for up to a year and a half after the initial menstrual TSS episode has gone away. I will give you a few quick examples. First, young women with menstrual TSS are likely to lose their hair in clumps during the disease and immediately upon recovery. This is distressing to say the least, but it is not permanent. As of today, we do not know why this happens. By the way, it also happens in other animals that develop TSS, so it is a shared, though not a life-threatening problem. Yes, other animals, including horses, dogs, cats, and even dolphins, develop TSS, even if such cases are not menstrual-related. Dolphins, for example, may develop *Staphylococcus aureus* infections of their blow-holes, leading to TSS and death.

Many patients ask: "Will I be able to get pregnant, or has this disease left me unable to have children?" There is no evidence that menstrual TSS alters ability to become pregnant and deliver normally.

The most discouraging delayed reaction after recovery is that many young women have serious memory lapses for up to one and a half years, forgetting important things, like where they are, why they are where they are, and with whom they are speaking. We do not know why this happens, ever since I started the major publicity on TSS back in 1980. I would think we would, but I guess it is being too hopeful for a disease described initially as affecting only women (cynically speaking). What is the biomedical science community thinking?

What do most high school seniors do to prepare for their futures? They take SAT and ACT entrance examination tests for college applications. This is difficult to do with serious memory lapses. Since I have helped with so many menstrual TSS cases, I can advise parents to ask for waiver of these exams, noting that their daughters' memories will return to "normal", hopefully by college time, and whatever "normal" means. I also remind all parents to be sure their daughters never ever use tampons again, to greatly reduce but not eliminate recurrences, even though recurrences may happen in absence of tampon use. Even today, we do not know why these recurrences happen in the absence of tampon use. I also advise parents to be sure their daughters get flu shots since TSS associated with influenza is highly fatal in young persons, reaching 100 percent fatal.[6] As noted previously but worth mentioning again, these young women will never develop immunity to the causative toxin (poison) because the toxin prevents that from happening.

How do you convince a parent, who has a daughter testing positive for herpes during TSS, that she is not sexually active? Believe your daughter! It's that simple. The positive test result is more likely than not simply to be a mistake. Some researchers originally and mistakenly thought that herpes virus was the cause of menstrual TSS.[7] However, immune system dysregulation, caused by the *Staphylococcus aureus* toxin (poison), results in this mistaken test result.

Thus overall, I become a sounding board for parents and physicians, hoping to offer my expertise freely as needed. Since I have consulted freely on so many TSS cases, I have significant accumulated knowledge. I will try throughout this book to convince you I have a reasonably good, long-term memory, and I am happy to help physicians and patients alike as requested. Now, let's move on.

As the book title says: What was I thinking? Here, I was in my first year—yes, very first year—as an Assistant Professor at the University of California, Los Angeles, (UCLA), having gotten a research grant from the National Institutes of Health to study a disease that reportedly did not exist. I described a toxin (poison), produced by the bacteria *Staphylococcus aureus*, that I knew was causing the disease, and that reportedly did not exist. I set up a required animal model to fulfill Koch's postulates (discussed later in this book) to show what causes the disease that reportedly did not exist. I even looked at environmental factors that controlled production of the toxin (poison) that caused the disease that reportedly did not exist. I was told by the biomedical science community and CDC for nearly two years that TSS did not exist. I knew the scoffers were wrong. The disease did exist, the toxin did cause the disease, the animal model was the correct one to study the disease, and the environmental factors that controlled production of the toxin (poison), later became important in showing why tampons were associated with this disease. So… what was I thinking? I was thinking that I was using grant money provided by American tax payers to study what I thought was an important disease, and that I owed my allegiance to the American public and not the biomedical science community. Thus, I spoke with a science writer on my thirty-first birthday, June 2, 1980, describing this disease to him and what caused it. The disease was menstrual toxic shock syndrome. The result of that discussion was an incredible nationwide news media storm that became second only in total news media coverage to the year-long Iran hostage crisis news coverage. The news attention to menstrual TSS was absolutely critical in advancing our understanding of all aspects of the disease, both menstrual cases and non-menstrual cases.

Menstrual TSS, as reported in June 1980, is a disease characterized by high fever (greater than 102°F), significant drop in blood pressure (systolic [the top number]) blood pressure of <90 millimeters of mercury), and a variable component usually seen as rapidly progressive flu-like symptoms, with vomiting and diarrhea being most common. The patients often have a fleeting sunburn-like rash. The disease is caused by *Staphylococcus aureus* secreting a toxin (poison called TSS Toxin) into the vagina of menstruating women. This toxin crosses the vaginal mucosa and leads to immune system dysregulation that manifests as TSS. When initially described, menstrual toxic shock syndrome killed 30 percent of patients.

This then is the story of what I can only describe as an amazing adventure in toxic shock syndrome, navigating the whims of the old-style CDC, and often, other biomedical scientists, putting up with too many sleepless nights, having many amazing and troubling discussions with scientists, and having a career working on behalf of those folks who supported my research. Do I have any regrets? With only a few exceptions, the answer is a grand NO! No regrets! Would I change anything? Yes! Among other things, I would ask our Congress definitely to make more funds consistently available to study diseases affecting women, diseases that even today are short-changed. This will become too obvious later in this book.

Folks also ask me all the time: "Who will read this book?" Good question! It is my hope that I have successfully straddled the now crumbling fence between what the American public will find interesting and what the biomedical scientific community will find as a complete update on toxic shock syndrome, and what remains to be understood.

As an aside, I do not want you to have to spend a lot of time reading footnotes. I personally find them very distracting. Thus, I will again add four references here that provide in-depth coverage of what I am saying in this book. If you want greater detail, refer to those scientific articles, and they in turn will refer you to many primary publications on the subject.[1,2,3,4] I will continue to provide references to some of the most important scientific publications.

Chapter 2

Gram–Positive Cocci: Really?

I need to say conclusively and many times throughout this book that toxic shock syndrome is caused by two kinds of bacteria: *Staphylococcus aureus* and *Streptococcus pyogenes*. Tampons are not the cause of TSS, but some have important co-causal roles in menstrual TSS. *Staphylococcus aureus* literally means circles of grape-like clusters that usually grow as gold-colored colonies on microbiology laboratory culture media. There are about ten million *Staphylococcus aureus* bacteria in a colony after overnight growth on laboratory media; about the size of a head of a pin. *Streptococcus pyogenes* means circles that grow in chains and induce pus (pyogenic). These are Latinized names of two closely-related bacteria which are exceptionally common causes of many kinds of human diseases, not to mention TSS.

I teach medical students, who are in training to become physicians, about both kinds of bacteria. I teach the students that *Staphylococcus aureus* are bacteria that are nearly always one micrometer in diameter, not able even to be seen unless magnified one thousand times by a microscope and even then, just barely so. To put this in perspective, it means that ten million of them can fit easily on the head of a pin. In other words, they are exceptionally tiny. However, only one is needed to cause human disease. Nearly 40 percent of us have the bacteria on our mucous membranes (nose, throat, intestinal tract, and genital tract) or skin at any given time, sometimes yes and sometimes no. We are nearly all genetically different, and because of this genetic diversity, we find that some persons always have the bacteria but some are intermittently infected. Why this is so is not known. Mostly, these *Staphylococcus aureus* bacteria do not cause us much trouble, except to cause us occasional painful boils, pimples, and maybe sinus infections. However, there are many kinds of *Staphylococcus aureus*. We scientists call these different varieties "many strains". The term, strain, is a loose term that allows scientists to define a bacterial strain with some special trait that we want to study, for example, the strain that produces a toxin called TSS Toxin-1, the cause of 100 percent of menstrual TSS. From here on, think of the causative toxin as TSS Toxin;[8] I will explain later why there is a "dash one" in the name that scientists use. Just remember that this is a potent poison, where the amount equal to a tenth of a grain of salt causes life-threatening TSS, and is secreted into humans by a unique strain of *Staphylococcus aureus*. At any given time, 5-10 percent of Americans have growing on mucous membranes or skin a strain that produces TSS Toxin. We call this being colonized by the bacteria on mucous membranes or skin. How this colonization with a TSS Toxin-producing strain affects humans is a major topic of this book. Many of us do not develop TSS because we have somehow developed immunity to TSS Toxin as we were growing up. Those who lack immunity may develop TSS.

I also tell medical students that *Staphylococcus aureus* can cause any disease that it wants to cause. It is by far the most significant cause of infections as noted in 2007 by the CDC.[9] Infections result in the greatest healthcare costs in hospitals in the United States, more than any other type of disease. *Staphylococcus aureus* infections lead to the greatest costs. Many of the decontamination processes, used in our hospitals to reduce the spread of infections, have been put in place to prevent *Staphylococcus aureus* transmission and infections.

Staphylococcus aureus are devils, as I can tell you from studying TSS and from my own personal experiences with staphylococcal infections. They turn our own immune systems against us to help them cause potentially serious infections. In addition to humans, other animals can be infected with the bacteria. For example, cows develop mastitis, udder infections, due to *Staphylococcus aureus*, causing the milking industry billions of dollars each year. The bacteria only cause infections in animals with immune systems, including then, all vertebrates. However, all groups of animals have their own kinds of *Staphylococcus aureus*. Thus, mainly human strains infect only humans, and animal strains infect only animals. There are occasional exceptions where this is not the case, and those strains can transiently cross species, usually to and from our pets and farm animals.

The kinds of *Staphylococcus aureus* infections range from pimples and boils to life-threatening bloodstream infections, infections of the heart, infections of the lungs, infections of bones, and infections of the kidneys. As I said above, the bacteria can cause whatever kinds of infections they want to cause in humans.

I remember a young man, twenty-five years of age, who had a serious automobile accident where he hit his head on the steering wheel. This head injury led to the surgical implantation of a metal plate under the skin of his forehead. In the course of the subsequent three days, and peaking on day five, the man developed the symptoms of TSS, including high fever, drop in blood pressure, and vomiting and diarrhea. He also developed a continuous, severe headache. The surgical site for implantation of the metal plate was surprisingly NOT highly inflamed, masking what was causing this TSS disease. Normally, infection sites would be expected to be inflamed, being red, swollen, warm, and painful. These are the four hallmark signs of inflammation. This, however, is not the case with infection due to TSS *Staphylococcus aureus*, where inflammation is often minor at worst. The man was placed on antibiotics and drugs to keep his blood pressure in the normal range, but these did not control the disease. On day five, the man said he felt like his head exploded, which essentially it did. Gross! What happened on day five was that the surgical site and implant were exploded out in a "pwock" sound, relieving pressure on his brain. The antibiotics then cleared the remaining bacteria, resulting in his recovery from both TSS and the severe headache. It turns out the man expelled (pwocked) nearly a cup of bacteria-filled liquid, without much pus, consistent with a lack of inflammation but including the metal plate. During initial implantation of the plate, skin *Staphylococcus aureus* had accidentally infected the site. The presence of any foreign body is well known by scientists to promote the ability of *Staphylococcus aureus* to grow in the site and cause disease. These bacteria are the bane of orthopedic surgeons, as 90 percent of bone infections are caused by *Staphylococcus aureus*. What do orthopedic surgeons do a lot of today? They implant artificial hips and knees by the thousands. If *Staphylococcus aureus* contaminate the implant site, the only thing that can be done in the following order is to remove the implant, then treat the infection, and then start over with implantation. The man is completely well today, and he has a new, non-infected metal plate implanted in his head. This case also makes an additional important point: males can develop toxic shock syndrome.

I am also reminded of a young woman who had knee replacement surgery. Over the course of the subsequent six months, she was variously diagnosed with rheumatic fever (autoimmunity), acute-onset rheumatoid arthritis (autoimmunity), systemic lupus erythematosus (autoimmunity), and behcets (autoimmunity). The diagnostic difficulties were the overlapping TSS symptoms with many diseases, the chronic nature of her disease, and the lack of inflammation; the incision site had completely healed over. Finally, a resident physician put a hypodermic needle in the healed-over surgical incision site and found he could withdraw a cup of plasma-like fluid that was full of TSS Toxin-producing *Staphylococcus aureus*. The woman thus had a variant form of toxic shock syndrome. The plasma-like fluid contained very few inflammatory cells. After withdrawal of the fluid and triple antibiotic therapy (vancomycin, clindamycin, and rifampin) and intravenous immunoglobulin, the patient recovered uneventfully.

I should add, it is never a good idea, from a patient point of view, to be a really interesting patient. I can say this from personal experience. These kinds of patients tend to have unusual clinical presentations, can be difficult to diagnose, and may lead to multiple case presentations, including in hospital grand rounds and in journal publications. She continues to be a real interesting case to present.

A woman elected to have an intraperitoneal implant to control unwanted urine discharge. The implant was placed through the vagina, and for some odd reason, as far as I am concerned, was implanted during her menstrual period. Unbeknownst to her and her surgeon, the woman had TSS Toxin-producing *Staphylococcus aureus* vaginally. She lacked antibodies to TSS Toxin. She of course developed menstrual TSS, which required removal of the implant and her being treated for TSS. She survived.

Since the early 1980s, I have published many times that 5-10 percent of women will have such bacteria present vaginally. Additionally, it has been known since the early 1980s that 20 percent of women will never develop protective antibodies against TSS Toxin.[10] Also, I have published many times, that if *Staphylococcus aureus* bacteria are present vaginally, the bacteria will be rare at times other than menstruation, kept in check by acid and hydrogen peroxide-producing lactobacilli; there may only be a few hundred *Staphylococcus aureus* bacteria. However, during menstruation, *Staphylococcus aureus* will grow vaginally from only a few hundred to one hundred billion, greatly increasing the chance of infection and TSS. Vaginal *Staphylococcus aureus* numbers peak on day two of menstruation because the vagina is no longer acidic but instead, is neutral in pH and contains lots of nutrients (food) for the bacteria to grow. This was the worst time to place the implant in this woman, and she did indeed develop TSS. Had she been tested first for vaginal *Staphylococcus aureus* producing TSS Toxin, and also tested second to see if she had antibodies to TSS Toxin, this surgery would not have been done, at least not until the bacterial numbers could first be reduced by antibiotics.

So, given all these kinds of cases, how are we protected from *Staphylococcus aureus* infections? Mostly, we are not protected from the bacteria themselves. However, by and large immunity depends on antibodies (immunoglobulins) that our immune systems make against the secreted toxins (poisons), including TSS Toxin. So... why do we not have vaccines against the infections? The reason is that by and large researchers have taken the wrong approaches. Researchers have wanted us to develop immunity against the staphylococci bacteria themselves instead of against the toxins. This is impossible with *Staphylococcus aureus*. I have published extensively on this subject in peer-reviewed scientific journals, showing that antibodies against the bacteria themselves cause the diseases in fact to be worse.[11] The bacteria clump in the presence of these antibodies, and *Staphylococcus aureus* bacteria like to clump to cause serious human diseases. Thus, antibodies against the bacteria themselves make the diseases more severe. For non-experts, all antibodies have two, four, or ten arms, and each arm with the ability to bind to and help cross-bridge two or more *Staphylococcus aureus* bacteria, ultimately resulting in clumps. Unfortunately, my predictions came true in a recent clinical trial where human patients were vaccinated or not vaccinated against the *Staphylococcus aureus* bacteria themselves but not the toxins. It turns out, in agreement with my expected findings, that five times as many persons, who were vaccinated, died compared to those not vaccinated.[12] This was definitely NOT a good vaccine. I had published my findings that such a vaccine would cause trouble, prior to this recent clinical study being done, yet the vaccine was a miserable failure. Why did this happen? Why was the clinical trial even done? What were they thinking? Certain groups of researchers, often those with "connections", get the most play, even if they are not doing the best science. Those scientists can choose to ignore prior data if it suits their needs. Very sad, but also very true.

Streptococcus pyogenes is the cause of the usual "strep throat", where there are millions of cases each year in the United States. Like *Staphylococcus aureus*, there are many strains of these bacteria. In August 1980, I told the CDC that these bacteria could cause streptococcal toxic shock syndrome, but it was not until 1987[13] and again in 1989[14] that I was able to publish clinical descriptions of this form of TSS in collaboration with my clinical colleagues (a.k.a. research physicians). When we published these descriptions, I should note that the fatality rate for streptococcal TSS at that time was nearly 85 percent, higher even than the scary Ebola Virus infections. Additionally, one-half of the survivors had limb amputations or had major parts of their bodies removed to save their lives. The disease became known as the flesh-eating streptococcal disease. This disease also killed the Muppeteer Jim Henson in 1989.

I started the publicity on this disease too, since again, there was strong resistance to recognition that the disease even existed. I could not begin publicizing the disease in 1980 because the news media and Federal Government, at that time, became so highly focused on staphylococcal TSS and its association with tampons that they simply were not hearing my concerns about streptococcal TSS; neither was the federal CDC. There may be as many as thirty-five thousand cases of the flesh-eating disease per year in the United States as I write today. I remember an investigator at the CDC saying to me: "Pat, if you had not publicized this disease in 1987 and again in 1989, we at the CDC would simply have ignored the disease. You dragged us into studying it, just like you did in 1980 with staphylococcal TSS."

I am comfortable with calling this the "flesh-eating" streptococcal disease. Some purist scientists are not comfortable since *Streptococcus pyogenes* bacteria do not have mouths and teeth for eating. However, this is just a human way of thinking, and *Streptococcus pyogenes* just goes about eating us in its own way. Think of it like this. The bacteria secrete toxins that liquify our tissues, making it into food. Then, it absorbs the liquified tissue (food), not through a single mouth but instead all throughout the cell. This greatly increases food intake per amount of time. This allows the bacteria to grow really fast, or as scientists say… exponentially. They double in numbers every forty-five minutes.

I have consulted on two thousand cases of streptococcal TSS, and I continue to do so today. I am reminded of the case of a woman who lost all four limbs (both arms and both legs) due to streptococcal TSS. This is in itself horrendous, but additionally she was a single mom with a newborn child. She clearly needed long-term care for both herself and her child. When I lost contact with the case, no longer being needed as a consultant, the woman's healthcare costs were already in the millions of dollars.

There was a young man in Wisconsin who was a weight-lifter, and one summer day he felt like he pulled a muscle in his left shoulder. That night, he developed a 102°F fever (normal body temperature is around 98.6°F). This 102°F fever is considered a high fever, and as I teach medical students, this is almost certainly a hallmark sign of bacterial infection. The man went to the emergency room at a local hospital where they thought he had heat prostration. They gave him an infusion in his arm of a liter (about a quart) of fluid since he also appeared dehydrated. The liter of fluid also cooled him down, so his body temperature came closer to normal. He then was released from the emergency room but remained sick with developing flu-like symptoms. What were they thinking? That night he developed a fever of 105°F and could not stand up; he was profoundly hypotensive, with very low blood pressure. He was rushed to the emergency room by his family, and there he had no blood pressure. The hospital staff was heroically able to restore his blood pressure to normal, and they brought his fever down. However, it was still completely unclear what was causing his symptoms. He had a mystery illness. The man went into a coma, and three months later, a physician on the case decided to stick a hypodermic needle into the shoulder muscle. He had noted, that in the first emergency room visit, the man complained that he may have pulled a shoulder muscle. The patient had self-medicated with non-steroidal anti-inflammatory agents (for example aspirin and ibuprofen), and this was masking excessive shoulder pain. As you now should expect, the physician pulled out of the site plasma-like fluid, without pus. The fluid was full of *Streptococcus pyogenes* and a TSS Toxin that caused his disease. The patient had streptococcal TSS with extensive muscle damage. In the end, the man woke up from his coma but only after surgical removal of most of his left back, left shoulder, and left chest muscles. He had what we now call streptococcal TSS with necrotizing myositis (infection of the muscle). He is very lucky to be alive today since that disease is nearly always fatal. We do not know even today why he lapsed into a coma, and why he later came out of the coma. I suspect it is because the causative toxin, Scarlet Fever Toxin A (related to TSS Toxin), was affecting his brain to cause the coma, and only after the toxin was removed, could the patient come out of the coma.

Let's move on. Toxic shock syndrome is the first disease, described over a period of forty years, in which the American public learned about the infection and disease real-time, just as investigators and physicians at the same time were learning about the disease. Along the way, many sad and sadly-humorous statements were made which I think portray the unfortunate current state of American scientific investigation. As my friend Dr. Roger Stone once said to me: "Research universities have much more political intrigue than any corporation has. However, we are always taught that the reverse is true."

I have quickly come to realize that Roger was correct. For example, this book is about TSS that includes the important tampon-associated menstrual disease. There have been lots of discussions, many times with little or no scientific data, as to why tampons are associated with menstrual TSS. In February 1983, I published what has become the primary "reason" tampons are associated.[15] That is, tampons according to absorbency bring in air (oxygen) into the normally anaerobic (without air) human vaginal environment. The highest absorbency tampons bring in more oxygen than low absorbency tampons. Oxygen is absolutely required for TSS Toxin to be produced by the bacteria *Staphylococcus aureus*. The toxin, once made, crosses the vaginal mucosa and sets off a cascade of dysfunctional immune system events that result in high fever, significant drop in blood pressure due to blood vessel leak, and many times a sunburn-like rash.

As an example of what I mean by having "little science" yet lots of opinion on TSS, I give the following example. Soon after I had published my studies on why tampons were associated with menstrual TSS, another university-based research group opined in the news that disposable diapers, with highly absorbent materials, were likewise associated with toxic shock syndrome, simply because of the presence of the highly absorbent fibers. I was at the forefront of news media publicity on TSS, as I had started the publicity to make the American public aware of the disease. Thus, I was asked for my opinion on the possible association with disposable diapers. I made two statements. First, I knew of absolutely zero, no cases of TSS associated with disposable diapers; I said: "Ask that research group to identify any such cases." Second, *Staphylococcus aureus* requires very specific conditions that will lead to production of the toxin that causes toxic shock syndrome, and those conditions are not present in disposable diapers, whether or not they are newly worn or soiled. The news media called the other research group, and the researchers admitted there had been no cases associated with disposable diapers. This ended that discussion, indeed as it should have. The real question, appropriately cynically, that should be asked is: "Why did this come up at all based on zero data?" I know the answer: to gain media attention. Later in this book, I will give many wrong-headed opinions that were put forward as to why tampons "caused" menstrual TSS, mostly put forward with no data.

In determination of whether a microorganism, such as *Staphylococcus aureus*, causes a disease, scientists are expected to fulfill a set of four criteria called Koch's postulates named after the German scientist Dr. Robert Koch. These postulates are set up linearly but sometimes as a circular chain, like a bracelet. The scientific community is expected first to fulfill them in order. The first postulate is to have a collection of symptoms that define a disease, with isolation of the proposed causative bacteria. We have that in toxic shock syndrome, as proposed by Dr. James Todd, Children's Hospital of Denver; this is the important, first and so-called clinical component of the chain.[16] Then, the chain continues such that there should be an association of the symptoms with a causative microorganism and its toxin, in this case *Staphylococcus aureus* that produces a toxin called TSS Toxin. It was not until 1981 that my research group published the causative TSS Toxin.[8] Large groups of investigators were also studying the association of TSS with menstruation and tampons, particularly with high-absorbency tampons. This is what is called the epidemiology of TSS, or what the risk factors are that lead to TSS.

The second of Koch's postulates is to isolate the proposed causative bacteria in pure form. This is a trivial exercise for isolation of *Staphylococcus aureus*, but this is not so trivial in identifying the causative toxin as will be explained in detail in a later chapter.

Subsequent to this, the third of Koch's postulates is that an animal model should be established that duplicates the disease. In 1981 in the *Journal of Infectious Diseases*, I established toxic shock syndrome in an animal model and re-isolated the causative bacteria, the microbiology component of the chain, fulfilling the last two criteria of Koch's postulates.[8]

Finally, the chain may continue back to assess clinically if there are variant forms of the disease to find the full expanse of clinical disease. If there are variants, the chain continues again with epidemiology, followed by microbiology.

There were many studies of the tampon association, including clinical description, epidemiology association with tampon use, and microbiology explanation for disease and tampon association. However, there has never been a clinical association with disposable diapers, there has never been an epidemiology association with disposable diapers, and finally, there are no microbiology data to support clinical or epidemiology with disposable diapers. Thus, I told the media this was chasing a "red herring", and it was likely done only to gain media attention. I have often stated that the scientific community should: "contaminate their non-scientific opinions in the news, first with scientific data." Many scientists do not like me saying this, but it is true. Today, often the surest way to believe you can gain grant support is to have something profound to say, including in the news media, particularly if you are well known and from a large, well-connected university.

Soon after menstrual toxic shock syndrome was described, I pointed out in the news media that cases occur in other individuals, such as children following influenza infection. I was told, particularly by members of the CDC, that this was not the case. A year and a half later, the CDC published on non-menstrual TSS. In 1987, the Minnesota Department of Health and I published a landmark paper describing post-influenza toxic shock syndrome.[6] Today, as I look at the data from that study, and carry the data forward up to today, when TSS Toxin-producing *Staphylococcus aureus* are present, the cases are 100 percent fatal—yes, 100 percent fatal. We also now know that other toxins, related to TSS Toxin, may cause post-influenza toxic shock syndrome; in such cases the patients may or may not die. Post-influenza TSS may be the most common form of the disease. So, as of my writing these words, the CDC notes, as printed in our local newspaper, that twenty-five children in the United States this year have died of influenza. I ask, is that what they died from, or did they die of secondary bacterial infections, such as TSS? Other kinds of non-menstrual TSS occur. For example, patients with nasal surgery develop TSS, so do patients with damaged skin, such as cold sores, surgical site infections, Darier White syndrome, and you name it *Staphylococcus aureus* infection. Of particular significance to me today is TSS Toxin-producing *Staphylococcus aureus* which are also highly associated with bullous pemphigoid, a blistering skin disease of the elderly, and eczema herpeticum, where patients have both herpes virus and *Staphylococcus aureus* skin infections. Both of these conditions can be fatal. Finally, there is another variant form of TSS, that we named extreme pyrexia syndrome.[17] Patients, for some unknown reason, respond with extreme fevers of 108°F in one hour, and their brains "fry" so fast that all of the patients so far described die due to the infection. I have not figured out a way to keep these patients alive.

Then we have streptococcal toxic shock syndrome caused by *Streptococcus pyogenes* (Group A streptococcus). This bacterium is commonly thought of as the cause of "strep throat", and that is true. However, in 1987 and 1989 with my clinical colleagues, we described emergent cases of streptococcal toxic shock syndrome in the *New England Journal of Medicine.* This again set off an appropriate news media blitz. My colleagues and I were on nearly all news media in the world. I did a fifteen-minute segment on the news show *20/20* one week after the historic slow Bronco drive on television by OJ Simpson. As I said, this streptococcal TSS became known as the flesh-eating streptococcal disease. The fatality rate when described was near 85 percent. With recognition and development of better treatments, the fatality rate dropped to near 30 percent. However, for reasons discussed later in this book, the fatality rate today for streptococcal TSS may be back up to 60 percent.

So, readers, I hope you continue and enjoy your trip through toxic shock syndrome. I trust you will come away with a great appreciation for the wandering path it took to unravel this disease. Finally, I hope you will see that scientists are not so different from other folks; their ivory towers are really not made of ivory. These folks should spend their time making the American public aware of what they are doing to benefit the public.

Chapter 3

A Small-Town Kid From Iowa;
Is That Anywhere Near Idaho?

I present this third chapter so that you will know who I am, and that with enough perseverance, economically poor folks like I was can make it in American society, even though it may be difficult and a very trying experience. I think I made it. This chapter sets the stage for why I was able to do what I did related to toxic shock syndrome—that is, risk everything to make the American public aware of a new disease in real time.

This is indeed the first time the American public learned about and was updated constantly about a disease at the same time as the scientific and medical communities learned and were updated. I have no regrets about starting the news publicity, and indeed, I think all of us with funding from the National Institutes of Health have a responsibility to tell the American public what we are doing. After all, the American public are paying taxes to fund our research. I learned to reject the "norms" in my life, including rejection of the chronic, abusive alcoholism of my father, and the skewed practices of various aspects of the biomedical community.

I began working full time at age fourteen in a small-town grocery store. Most importantly, I learned to take risks to do what I felt was the right thing to do.

What did I have to lose? I had very little with which to begin. Essentially, I had to become an adult at fourteen years of age, so when I began the "publicity" on toxic shock syndrome in June of 1980, I already had been an adult-equivalent for seventeen years, making decisions that affected both my career and the American public.

So... who am I? I am a complete science nerd as I mentioned earlier. That's me through and through. I was voted most likely to become a nuclear physicist by my high school graduation class. What could be more nerdy than that? Look at what nerds the atomic physicists Albert Einstein, Max Planck, and Neils Bohr were. I grew up poor in small towns in North Central Iowa, Dakota City-Humboldt; these two towns are connected and separated from each other only by a set of railroad tracks. I guess I was on the wrong side of the tracks in Dakota City most of my young life. A principal once said to my older brother: "You Dakota City kids should be thankful we let you come to our fine high school in Humboldt." As if he had any say in where we went to school! The easiest thing for me to do without any money was to look for pretty rocks, mainly agates, geodes, and fossils, study stars and planets, make leaf collections, and grow microbes on Petri plates after school with my biology teacher, David Buffington, in the biology classroom.

I think my high school classmates saw me as a quiet but reasonably nice person, but because of my dismal family life, I had few true friends. It was impossible to invite anyone over to my home. One friend does stand out. He grew up with even less money than I did, if that's even possible. We used to play chess in the evening, and just talk about things. We played a few games at each get-together, but we decided to play best out of fifty to decide who was best. I think he bested me twenty-six to twenty-four. My friend had an unbelievably difficult childhood, but he rose above all the "crap" he had in front of him. I spoke to him a few years ago and continue interaction on *Facebook*, and I see now he is a minister; he has forgiven the many folks who tormented him, just for being poor. I remember one evening, when we left his room for a minute to help his sister, a neighborhood teenager came in and peed on his bed, soaking it completely through the mattress. There should be a special place in hell to deal with jerks like the neighbor teen. My friend is a better man than I will ever be in the years I have left.

As noted above, I started working full-time in a grocery store when I was fourteen years old; I remember my take-home pay was $20 per week. Most of that take-home money went for food and clothes for my younger brother and sister and me. I used to buy just-out-of-date meat to conserve money.

One thing I value in university life more than any other is faculty members who develop what I call appropriate cynicism. We need this to survive the administrative whims of universities as we try to perform our research, teaching, and service missions. I bring this up here to give you an early-year example of how you can develop cynicism.

While working at Hood's grocery store, making 85 cents an hour in 1964, one day a truck pulled away from the First National Bank across the street. It hit a bump, the back door popped opened, and a duffle bag of bank money bounced out. I saw this and immediately walked over, picked up the bag, and took it inside the bank to return it. The bank personnel thanked me, and that was it. Flash forward many years, where folks continuously have said I should have asked for 10 percent recovery fee for returning the found money. However, I thought returning the money simply was the right and responsible thing to do.

Now, consider this. While I was in college at the University of Iowa, I read a newspaper article about a financial advisor who had misappropriated and misspent $13 million of the same First National Bank's money, bankrupting the bank. Yes, it was the same bank as above, and this financial advisor's father was the bank president. This "bad actor" was one year ahead of me in Humboldt High School, being captain of nearly every team and most likely to succeed. His story made the news for several days, where the perpetrator had ultimately fled arrest, leaving his car in a parking lot at O'Hare Airport. The state governor at the time, Harold Hughes, convinced him to return and face up to his crime. The "perp" did in fact give himself up. It was interesting to find out in the news the sordid details of this escapade. For example, he had two complete families. The entire affair played out in the newspapers and on the radio. After completing his prison sentence, what did he do with his life? He went back to employment as a financial advisor, only now he had to have someone monitoring him closely. So, with nothing I return a bag of money, but a person with everything commits the crime of completely misusing the same money.

I want to give you an additional example of my life as a young kid of ten to fourteen. I did not have a bed on which to sleep. Instead, for those years, I slept on a ratty old couch when the weather was warm, and on a rug on the floor, with my older brother, in front of a fuel-oil stove with warm blower, during the winter. I shared the couch with a family of rats—yes, bona fide rats! I slept on the top, and they came in each evening to nest underneath. During the day, I could chase them into the cellar, which was a horror pit of mud, rat holes, and creepy stuff. Even horror writer Stephen King would have had trouble hanging out in our cellar. During the winter, my older brother and I had to walk two blocks, twice a day, to Odenbrett's Gas Station, to have a five-gallon container filled with fuel oil for heat. Unfortunately, we had to invert the container on the oil-burner stove, and fuel oil leaked onto the floor and into a rug we slept on. I have never been sure if the fuel oil fumes and fuel oil itself had harmful effects on our health. I remember one day Mrs. Odenbrett came to our house demanding payment for the fuel oil already charged. I paid this bill from my savings since my father had drunk up his paycheck.

When my father passed away, the minister commented that: "Bob was a terrible father." Imagine a minister saying that about anyone. To his credit, my father gave up both drinking and smoking after the four kids left home; mostly this was done because he was hospitalized for what he thought was a dread disease called "delirium tremens". I think he found out that this disease was caused by excessive drinking and that increased susceptibility to bloodstream infections could kill him. The minister at the funeral also added that: "Bob was a better grandfather."

When I was in high school, the guidance counselor met with students who he thought were going to college—that is, those who were college material. He did not choose to meet with me. It was not until one day the principal of the school, Mr. Delmar Cram, said to me: "Pat, you should decide on a college since your town of Dakota City is going to award you a scholarship based on you having the highest grade-point-average in your hometown." It was only then that I applied to attend the University of Iowa, the only place I applied; I also took the ACT test at that time. I scored 32 out of a 36 maximum possible score. I was accepted at the University of Iowa.

At high school graduation, while I was walking on stage to receive my diploma, the principal stopped the progression of events. He announced that I was also to be awarded a second, one year-scholarship provided by a family in Humboldt, as voted on by the teachers at the Humboldt-Dakota City High School. This money, plus a National Defense Education Act (NDEA) loan, allowed me to begin in the fall of 1967 as an undergraduate.

I was directed towards science as a major, just not exactly sure in which science I was most interested. I was assigned a geology professor Dr. Sherwood Tuttle (now deceased) as my advisor, and he worked with me to set up a plan as a geology major. Each year, I took required courses, such as rhetoric, literature, and social science cores, and then I also took courses in the sciences, mostly in geology but also chemistry and physics.

When I became a college senior, I began to think that the major geographic areas where you find interesting geology are places where you find few or no people: out in oceans, or in the arctic. My thinking was, *I am really interested in pretty rocks (gems) that are worth lots of money, and not geology per se.* This remains as true today as it was then. When I travel, I try to look for pretty rocks along the way. It was then that I began to enroll in biology courses, in addition to those courses required for geology. The one required course in geology that I did not take was a summer field course required for graduation with a geology bachelor's degree. Thus, my Bachelor of Arts (BA) degree in 1971 was in general science with emphasis in geology instead of strictly geology.

This was a BA degree and not a BS degree. This meant I also had to take two languages for graduation. My options for geology were French, German, Russian, and computer science. Because so many students were taking French and German, I took Russian and computer science. I also took scientific Russian, so I came to know cool words like кислород (pronounced Keesloroad), meaning oxygen. I can still read scientific Russian, almost fifty years later. I remember some computer science, Fortran, but who cares? I cannot speak Russian except single words or small phrases, and I am not fluent generally in computer science. I can use a computer!

Along the way, I worked as a geologist for two organizations, one a company and one the US Geological Survey. Although I mostly enjoyed the work, I was not really "amped up" by the work. I thus, again, applied to the University of Iowa to pursue a master's degree in science education, while I was redirecting my career. I was accepted and took courses towards this degree. However, I did a rotation in a junior high science classroom that completely turned me off to becoming a junior high or high school classroom teacher.

I was assigned to assist in what was referred to as the "dummy class", a class with a strong, engaging teacher, and who was assigned to teach introduction to physical sciences to seventh-grade "dummies". My experience was that I could not teach even basic physical science to these kids unless I could improve their math background. Many of the kids were functioning at a third to fourth-grade level, unable even to do fractions. I asked if I could help these kids with their mathematics, but immediately the parents of the kids became involved, and I was sternly shut down with: "How dare you think our kids do not know mathematics. What's the matter with you?" This more than convinced me to go in a different direction. Certainly, I was young and naïve, but I did not anticipate the exceptionally negative reaction from parents.

For a time, I went back to my comfort zone, working in a grocery store in Iowa City, by the name of Eagles, while I continued to redirect my future. I knew that although I was interested in the physical sciences, I was mostly interested in microbiology, as in what I had been doing in tenth-grade biology class. I made the most important and fulfilling decision in my career. I spoke with Dr. Allen Markovetz (now deceased), Director of Graduate Studies in the Microbiology Department at the University of Iowa. Soon after, I was accepted as a graduate student, doing thesis work on innate immunity.

On August 29, 1970 my wife and I became married. At that time, we both worked essentially at minimum wage. To show you what life was like for us, I present two examples. One, we lived in a one-bedroom apartment in Iowa City and could afford only $10 per week for groceries. We lived on precisely-divided-up, small portions of tuna and noodle casserole for most of my senior year of college and the following year. Two, we hitch-hiked to many places we needed to go. Our car was in the shop for much of the time. I walked five miles each morning to the Eagles grocery store and five miles home after work. Occasionally, the Iowa City police would give me a ride, much appreciated, since I was walking at 5:00 A.M.

I think they were worried initially that I was up to "no-good", but they then realized that I was simply walking a long way to work. This long walk gave me a lot of time to think about my future. Also, geologists spend a lot of time looking down, searching for rocks. This meant I found lots of things, including watches, other jewelry, and money. I would turn the valuable things I found in to the police, except money, and most were returned to me after a year, as unclaimed. My spouse worked for the Iowa Testing Program at the University of Iowa. This group was responsible for the well-known Iowa Basic Skills Test (also known as Iowa Test of Educational Development).

My wife and I have one daughter who is one of the brightest persons I know.

For a time, as noted above, I worked for a company as a geologist. I had collected a sludge-pile of dense, discard junk that could not be used in commercial sand. The mined sand from Waterloo, Iowa, was shot up into the air with water and dense material, which did not go up, collected in this sludge pile. The sand would blow into a different pile. I was given permission by the company to have the sludge. In the evening, I would sit at the Iowa City Park and pan the sludge for gold. Gold, scraped down to Iowa by glaciers, was indeed present in the dense sludge. Over time, I found eight small gold nuggets, which I still have, and which are worth about $3,000. Most importantly, I found an old quarter, which when cleaned up I immediately sold for $40. It was valued at $75, but we needed the money, so $40 was perfectly fine. I should also note that the neighborhood kids, usually ages seven to ten, with their parents, would come to watch me pan for gold. I would often times show them how to pan. They were excited by finding a few grains of gold fleck. This showed me something that is even true today. Kids about seven to ten years of age seem to like me. The most interesting thing about young kids is that they do not have hidden agendas, unlike many adults I have encountered.

I have always thought I might have been the poorest (in monetary terms) student at the University of Iowa. When I left my hometown to come to the university, without my parents' help or encouragement, all of my belongings fit in a box one by one by three feet; this included two pairs of blue jeans ($6 each from Degroote's Clothing Store), three t-shirts ($5 each and one a hand-me-down from my older brother), and underwear and socks. The tennis shoes I had on were the total for shoes. I lived in Hillcrest Dormitory, which still functions as a dorm today.

My next-door neighbors in the dorm were two scholarship football players: quarterback Ed Podolak and running back Kerry Reardon, both of whom went on to play pro-football in Kansas City. Wow, did they have clothes; more than a closet-full. Clearly, they were well off. I also remember walking by the Black Student Union, which was occupied by many football players. I kept thinking how well off they were compared to me. I now know that the large majority of African Americans were poor. I was the first person in my family to go to college. Today, we would consider me as part of a protected class of students, comparable to under-represented minorities, but this was not the case back in my college days.

I spent $1,492 my freshman year. This covered tuition, room and board, except no dinner on Sundays, and the cost of books and supplies. I worked in the Hillcrest Dining Room my freshman year, cleaning the floors after lunch and dinner. My major job was mopping because the football players had their meals in Hillcrest and often had food fights. The rest of us in the dorm never ate as well as the football players.

My sophomore year is also worth mentioning. Because of never having dinner on Sunday my freshman year, I vowed to do things differently my sophomore year. I lived in approved, off-campus housing. I spent $860 my sophomore year. I raised acorn squash the summer preceding my sophomore year, and I had one acorn squash every day with a small amount of hamburger, except the last two weeks of school. It was those last two weeks that I had only Harvest Day (store brand; 8 cents a can) tomato soup with water for breakfast, lunch, and dinner. I am six feet tall, and I lost weight to 140 pounds; I was becoming a waif.

I received financial aid scholarships for my junior and senior years, and these helped tremendously. I also took advantage of National Defense Education Act loans and specific loans to geology majors from an endowment. These, I have long since repaid.

One funny thing happened my sophomore year. I was studying calculus on a Friday night. My three roommates had gone out to have fun. I had my feet up on a small table when the apartment was hit with an earthquake. Pretty cool for a geology major! This earthquake left a one-inch gap the entire length of the apartment.

I have a pretty good memory. My biology teacher, who had long-since moved to teach in Connecticut, called me out of the blue a few years ago when he was preparing to retire. He had found some news clips about me and toxic shock syndrome. He asked out of the blue: "Who is the best-looking person you know?" I had not spoken with David since my tenth-grade biology class.

My immediate response was: "Next to me, it must be you." He then asked if I knew who was calling. I knew, even though we had not spoken for nearly fifty-five years. I say this so that you will know the stories that follow this are true to the best of my knowledge and memory, which I think is pretty good. Along this line also, folks often ask me where to find articles on toxic shock syndrome, for example autopsy data. I immediately answer: "Volume 96, 1982 *Annals of Internal Medicine*."[18] As I say, I am a complete science nerd through-and-through. Ask me to remember people's names, and I have trouble. So, maybe I am more of a savant with intense knowledge in math and science.

After graduation with a PhD degree in microbiology, and specifically innate immunity, in 1976 I signed on for three more years (1976-1979) of training, called postdoctoral training, at the University of Minnesota, Department of Microbiology. My mentor was the Department Chair Dr. Dennis Watson (now deceased). He allowed me to run his laboratory, and I trust he knew just how incredibly important this was to me and my career. It was during this time, to be discussed in more detail later, that I became aware of toxic shock syndrome. In Dennis's laboratory I was studying streptococcal scarlet fever; his laboratory was the most expert laboratory in the world studying the toxins (poisons) that cause scarlet fever. It turns out the scarlet fever toxins are related to TSS Toxin.

Chapter 4

What do Research Faculty do Anyway Besides Sit in Ivory Towers?

I have been a faculty member since 1979 at three large public universities, University of California, Los Angeles (UCLA); University of Minnesota; and University of Iowa. I am old now at seventy years old. I am proud to say that I have never been at one of the United States large private universities. Public universities have the reputation, with which I agree completely, as bringing the largest number of folks out of poverty. On a recent National Public Radio show, it was shown that State University of New York, Stony Brook is the public university with the greatest ability to bring poor students out of poverty. In contrast, it has been demonstrated that Washington University, St. Louis, MO, a private university, is the university with the worst reputation of helping low-income people out of poverty (This presentation is summarized at the following site: https://www.northernpublicradio.org/post/are-colleges-helping-americans-move.) This of course means that some faculty members at the large private universities have told me, essentially, I am a "dumb shit"—dumb for remaining at a public university and thus, too dumb to discover anything new, I presume. Yes, as I said, some of these folks have let me know in no uncertain terms how smart-less I am. I say this with cynicism. You may agree with them, but I would argue that you have not read long enough in this book to know for sure... so please read on, and then make your decision. You may let me know at patrick-schlievert@uiowa.edu.

As a faculty member at public universities, I have had three roles: 1) do research or as we sometimes call it perform scholarship; 2) teach; and 3) perform public service. It is clear to me and many others that public universities are the greatest thing in post-high school education, especially after World War II. With the GI Bill and National Defense Education Act loans, many returning veterans, and kids like me, could get a post-high school degree and in this way be of service to our country. Indeed, our local paper this morning (January 2020) tells me that an independent research group has shown that the Iowa Regents' Universities, through their education missions, enhance the state by $11.8 billion per year (Please see this website: https://www.thegazette.com/subject/news/education/ regent-research-finds-118-billion-impact-in-iowa-by-states-public-universities-20191114). This means a return on investment of nearly four dollars for each dollar invested in the universities. Through National Defense Education Act loans, I was able to obtain a bachelor's degree from the University of Iowa in 1971. I then received a PhD degree in microbiology and immunology in 1976 through research assistantships from grants held by my mentors. Because I remained in a public institution of higher education, one-half of my federal National Defense Education Act loans were forgiven. My tuition at the University of Iowa in 1967-1971 was $240, $260, $320, and $370 per year. Plus, I lived on campus my freshman year as required at that time and incurred debt by doing so, so my entire National Defense Education Act borrowing was $2,600 for the four years. I was only required to pay back $1,300. Today, students pay $8,000 in tuition per year at the University of Iowa. Like so many other public universities, they are starved for support by state legislatures who have forgotten how legislators benefitted from these public universities. When Ronald Reagan was president, he eliminated the National Defense Education Act loan system. Major bummer!

As a faculty member at public universities, and at each one, I have taught microbiology and immunology to an enormous number of students. For example, in the thirty-one years I was at the University of Minnesota, I taught microbiology and immunology to one-third of all physicians-in-training, those are medical students, ever trained at the university since its inception. I also taught medical students at

UCLA and the University of Iowa, just not the same number as at Minnesota, since I was not at these two universities for the same long period of time. While at Minnesota, I also taught microbiology and immunology to undergraduates, 260 per year for five years. I have likewise trained twenty-seven graduate students, all of whom have become the next generation of educators and researchers, both in university settings and industry. I am very proud of this teaching accomplishment which is usually deemphasized at large private universities.

A few years ago, I was told by faculty members at one large East Coast private university that: "Teaching is for those faculty members who cannot obtain National Institutes of Health grant funding for research." I have never felt this way, likely because I grew up poor as dirt and was happy to have wonderful professors at the University of Iowa from 1967-1976. It was amazing to me how smart these Iowa faculty members were, and all I could do is try to pattern myself after them. I hope I have lived up to their standards. I pattern my teaching style after Dr. George Becker (now deceased), and I pattern my research enthusiasm after Drs. Rudy Galask, Bill Johnson, and Al Markovetz. I have received multiple teaching awards voted on for separate awards by medical students (eight total), medical school faculty (only one allowed), university faculty (only one allowed), and the major society I belong to… the American Society for Microbiology (only one allowed). I retired my name from consideration for awards voted on by medical students since there are many other terrific faculty members who merit recognition. I have never regretted spending a major part of my life teaching.

I am likely to be in the great minority in the next set of comments on our research in the United States. All you need to do is look at the Blue Ridge Institute for Medical Research to see that the top universities in National Institutes of Health granted funding primarily are large private universities, and not the large public universities. Why is this? There are several reasons. Historically, these private universities have hired assistant professor faculty members, often with no intent to promote them to associate professors with tenure. This allows them to set standards that each faculty member must have three to four research grants, and with these funds, the assistant professors must pay their salaries as well as do research. Importantly, they must pay high indirect costs. Indirect costs refer to money needed to keep the lights on. This should be relatively the same at all universities, but indirect costs can vary greatly, with indirect costs typically much higher at private universities. Note, I also said, the private universities typically pay very little of the salaries of the assistant professors. Additionally, many of the assistant professors cannot maintain three to four research grants, and they must leave after six to eight years, usually taking their one to two grants with them to public universities. In contrast, assistant professors at public universities are expected to gain at least one research grant, where the indirect costs are also lower. At the same time, these public university faculty members are expected to teach in order to qualify for promotion to associate professor with tenure. Generally, if the assistant professors at public universities have one to two grants, do a good job of teaching, and perform service to the community, they receive promotion to associate professor status with tenure.

What does it mean to have tenure? After spending six to eight years as assistant professors, faculty members who do their jobs will be promoted to associate professors with what is called indefinite tenure. Indefinite tenure is granted so faculty members cannot easily be terminated. This is done to allow faculty to change research areas without penalty, to teach courses that may be controversial, and to help the community in terms of service without penalty. This is what we want faculty members to do, and this is the reason public universities are so important.

A tenured physics professor at the University of Minnesota was doing an excellent job of teaching physics. However, he decided that he also wanted to teach a course in communism. Because of this, the university president attempted to terminate the faculty member. The president was not allowed to do this, nor should he be allowed to do so. It should be okay for a faculty member to teach a course to acquaint students with what life is like in communism, even if this is unpopular. Universities should not stick their heads in the sand.

I am also reminded that many university presidents and outside legislators ask why we continue to teach geography in colleges. Who needs it? The thought is that we all know the entire geography of the world. So, why teach geography? I think of a UCLA faculty member asking the entire microbiology and immunology department to find Iowa on a blank United States map. Only the original Iowans could do this. If geography is so unimportant that we do not need to teach geography, then all folks should minimally know where the states are in their own country.

Now, I ask where is the Crimea, and what do we know about the people in Crimea? Most folks in the United States likely cannot answer either part of that question, but both are critical aspects of geography, and our dealings with both the Ukraine and Russia.

I want to go back to public versus private universities. In elementary through high school, we only allow public funds to be used to educate students in public schools. Students in private schools must pay tuition, separate from public funds. So, why do we not infuse more money into public universities, through both legislatures and through the National Institutes of Health, and at the expense of funding going to large private universities? I pay taxes, not so private universities can mistreat assistant professors. Instead, I pay taxes so public universities can thrive, both in their teaching mission and in doing the critical research for our country. To a small extent Congress is addressing this by establishing COBRE states, states underrepresented in National Institutes of Health research grant funding. The problem is there are a myriad of public universities who do not qualify for COBRE funding.

You may disagree with me on public versus private university funding for research. You may say: "What we want is high-quality research, regardless of who is doing it." This would be acceptable to me if indeed researchers at large private universities always had the American public's interest in mind. I question whether this is generally happening. Also, research importance is in the eye of the beholder. I mention later that tuberculosis and breast cancer research were at one time tremendously underfunded. Indeed, Dr. Patrick Brennan at the Colorado State University was the only person funded to do research on tuberculosis until Congress mandated additional funding. One person in seven who dies in the world dies of tuberculosis. My Uncle Charles developed tuberculosis from fighting in the South Pacific during World War II. At that time, there were no effective antibiotics. Today, we are verging again on not having antibiotics due to resistance.

I recently saw an enormous research program at a large private university funded to study the role of antibodies in immunity to tuberculosis. There is no role for antibodies in immunity to tuberculosis that I can see! I think the data are completely clear that not antibodies, but instead CD4 T lymphocytes activating macrophages are responsible for immunity. It is important not that you know the difference between antibodies and CD4 T lymphocytes activating macrophages but only that you know they are very different in what they do. But, gee whiz, those researchers at the private university are noted as doing such "elegant research". I am of the opinion that elegance is not what we want. What we want is what the American public can hang its hat on, or if not Americans, then the world. There is a tuberculosis vaccine that is used in many parts of the world. It is by no means perfect. However, it works well enough that many countries are using it. It just needs to be perfected. The vaccine stimulates protective CD4 T lymphocytes activating macrophages.

Some private universities are now offering free tuition to medical students. They have such large endowments that they can afford to do so. Public universities cannot do this. Where did those large endowments come from? Were they at the expense of money coming to public universities? I think the answer is in part… yes.

This does not mean that I am a complete curmudgeon relative to private universities. It is just that we need to do some readjusting to make things equitable. Some of my former students are at large private universities, and they are doing well. Sorry friends, but I am entitled to my own ridiculous opinion on this subject.

Chapter 5

In the Beginning Microbiology and Immunology Were Created and Invaded and Subdued Medicine

You think the title of this chapter is wrong? Just watch television for a short period of time, and you will see so many commercials, maybe half, are advertising monoclonal antibodies that block immune system function. These antibodies are used for management of rheumatoid arthritis, psoriasis, inflammatory bowel disease, and many other conditions. Warnings include being aware of infections that may occur.

I should take a few minutes to explain microbiology and immunology from my perspective, as related to human diseases. Microbiology is the study of bacteria, viruses, fungi, and parasites, which cause human diseases; there are many other areas of microbiology, for example industrial, but I will not address these in any detail. However, I hope you are having wine or beer, as a result of yeast fermentation, as you read this book.

Here is a funny occurrence that happened when I was a faculty member in microbiology and immunology at the University of Minnesota. Each year all faculty members in the university who do microbiology research are required to update their training in how to handle infectious microorganisms. The university upper administration saw that was a tedious process. It was also exceptionally costly in terms of faculty time. Thus, the upper administration decided to hire and bring in a public health official from the University of California, Davis to present the update, in three sessions, to all faculty members who required such training. Seems like a good idea… am I correct? Get the training done efficiently.

Please remember that a very large number of the trainees (faculty members) were microbiologists studying infectious, pathogenic microorganisms. They all had doctorate degrees, combinations of PhD, MD, and MD/PhD degrees. The person doing the training was known to have a master's degree in public health. This made the session introduction interesting.

The trainer started by telling all of us in the audience that there are five major classes of microorganisms that cause disease. My immediate thought, and the thinking of my neighbor trainees, was that there are only four classes of microorganisms, so this would be interesting to see what the new category is. The trainer defined the five classes: 1) bacteria, 2) viruses, 3) fungi, 4) parasites, and the brand new one 5) rickettsia. At this point most trainees tuned out. Rickettsia are kinds of bacteria, so indeed there are only four major kinds, as we originally thought.

The trainer went on to explain that we may have had grant funding from the National Institutes of Health to study development of a vaccine against hepatitis C virus. If you watch TV for any period of time, you will know that there is a treatment for hepatitis C virus infections, but this treatment is costly. A vaccine would be exceptionally helpful. We already have approved and used vaccines against hepatitis A and B viral infections. Incidentally, hepatitis means that the viral infection is damaging a vital organ, the liver. These infections can lead to fatal bloodstream secondary infections and cancers. So, what did the trainer say next? He emphasized that indeed we may have had funding from the National Institutes of Health to study hepatitis C virus vaccine development, but continued to say: "However, there is no current vaccine against this virus, so the University Biosafety Committee has the right to tell you that you cannot do research to develop a vaccine against hepatitis C virus, but you should use the funding to do research on hepatitis B virus, since there is an existing vaccine." What was he thinking? There are two things wrong with this thinking: 1) you have funding to develop a hepatitis C virus vaccine, and you are not allowed by the National Institutes of Health to use the funding for a very different purpose; and 2) we already have a hepatitis B virus vaccine, and we need a vaccine against hepatitis C virus. It simply makes no sense at all to redevelop a hepatitis B virus vaccine. The current vaccine against hepatitis B virus is highly effective. You could argue that hepatitis C virus is too dangerous to allow microbiologists to study. I would point out that we are very highly trained in the safe handling of infectious microbes. Indeed, I have friends who research HIV/AIDS, Ebola virus, and flesh-eating streptococcal disease, all of which I would argue are more dangerous than hepatitis C virus. In the end, most of us did not listen to the trainer. I should also note that I was the trainer for medical students for teaching blood-borne pathogens, including hepatitis viruses. However, someone else, like the person from the University of California, Davis, had to train me. I could not train myself. There is just something "wrong-headed" with this thinking. I am good enough to train medical students, but I am not sufficiently trained to provide training to such an important group. Yes... you could argue that I could use additional training, just in case. Then, be sure the person doing the update is not the above person from California.

The next few paragraphs discuss the real four kinds of microbes that cause human diseases. This is not comprehensive, but it gives you a representative picture.

The bacterium *Staphylococcus aureus* causes boils, pimples, and other soft tissue infections, making it the most common cause of infectious diseases. Those same bacteria cause seventy thousand cases of pneumonia each year in the United States, with a 60 percent fatality rate, forty thousand cases of infections of the heart, known as infective endocarditis, and thus forty thousand cases of bloodstream infections, both with a 40 percent fatality rate. The same bacterium causes over five hundred thousand cases of surgical site infections in hospitals and causes infections in over thirty million Americans with diabetes and an additional thirty million with eczema (atopic dermatitis). Finally, the bacteria are the most common causes of bone infections, known as osteomyelitis. Why do people die from *Staphylococcus aureus* infections? There are many strains or varieties of *Staphylococcus aureus*, and all that cause disease in humans produce one or more potent poisons (toxins) that kill people. This bacterium and its potent toxins are major subjects of this book.

We have all heard of antibiotics. The vast majority of antibiotics have bacteria as their targets. The reason is that bacteria are very different from us. This means we can find antibiotics that will kill bacteria and not us because of those differences. For example, there are a lot of penicillin antibiotics. Penicillins all prevent bacteria from growing by preventing production of a required cell wall around bacteria. Human cells do not have cell walls around them.

Most of the antibiotics in use came originally from fungi (examples: *Penicillium* and *Cephalosporium*) or other bacteria (example: *Streptomyces*) that live in the soil and use these antibiotics to create space in the soil for them to grow. Humans have now made many modifications to the antibiotics, but even with those new modifications, we are on the verge of losing ability to fight bacteria. Bacteria, like *Staphylococcus aureus*, can grow in humans to very high levels, for example, up to one hundred billion in the vagina of women during menstruation. It turns out that about 1 bacterium in a million is a mutant, so in the human vagina there may be one hundred thousand mutants, some of which become resistant to new antibiotics. This is why hospitals and medical clinics are supposed to be careful in antibiotic use... so we do not select for antibiotic resistance in bacteria, and then lose ability to treat infections. As an aside: If you let bread sit, it will become moldy, usually with a blue-green mold (molds are fungi). If you place the moldy bread in a Ziploc® bag with water to keep it humid, in a few days a yellow liquid may appear on the surface of the mold. That yellow liquid is penicillin produced by the *Penicillium* mold.

Viruses also cause human diseases, for example measles, mumps, German (three-day) measles, hepatitis, Acquired Immunodeficiency Syndrome (HIV/AIDS), COVID-19, and influenza. I mention influenza last since this virus commonly causes respiratory infections, some of which are secondarily infected with *Staphylococcus aureus*, which become life-threatening pneumonia. We are only now asking if the same kinds of secondary infections occur after COVID-19. I am sure the answer is yes.

We speak of the 1918 worldwide pandemic of influenza that killed two million Americans and millions of folks in other countries. These persons rarely died as a result of influenza, but instead they died of secondary bacterial infections due to *Streptococcus pneumoniae*, *Haemophilus influenzae*, and

Staphylococcus aureus. When I first proposed this notion, it was not accepted, and maybe it is not universally accepted today. However, I first made the statement at a review of the National Institutes of Health Rocky Mountain Laboratories for which I was on a review panel. The director of the National Institutes of Allergy and Infectious Diseases, Dr. Anthony Fauci, had given a terrific seminar on how influenza infections have become less fatal over the years, largely from improved medical care. I agree with him! However, we disagreed on why folks were dying in the first place. The Spanish Flu of 1918 coincided with the end of World War I, and many returning soldiers were run-down and starving as a result of the war... the perfect individuals to develop serious influenza infections, with secondary bacterial infections to kill them. It is interesting that several months later Dr. Fauci published a paper in which he showed that you could hardly find evidence of influenza infections in tissues from the 1918 influenza pandemic, but there was ample evidence to indicate the folks died of secondary bacterial infections.[19] One of my common statements to medical students is: "Viruses often use bacteria to do their dirty work, such as killing people." An easy way to tell the difference, between influenza alone and influenza with a secondary bacterial infection, is fever. Again, I remind medical students that most viruses cause infections with fevers, peaking at around 101°F or lower. However, serious bacteria super-infections of influenza often have fevers in excess of 103°F. Typically, children with influenza will have a fever for a few days and then begin to recover. If, however, they become secondarily infected with *Staphylococcus aureus* producing TSS Toxin, they will develop a new fever as high as 108°F, and 100 percent will die as a result of dramatic drop in blood pressure or severe brain damage as a result of fever. I will address this in more detail later. Yes, I said 100 percent could die. Why? The answer is that the disease progression may be too fast for physicians to recognize and respond. However, physicians and microbiologists are also often compartmentalized to think one microbe causes one disease. This means influenza virus is recorded as causing all influenza, including fatal cases, even though bacteria are doing the virus's dirty work to kill the patients. It is possible that the fatality rate may not be 100 percent if physicians automatically think *Staphylococcus aureus* and possibly other bacteria when they think influenza.

My friend Dr. Arturo Casadeval reminds me that fungi are the major genocide experts in the world. I remind him that this is only because fungi have not learned to cause disease without killing everything. When I say everything, I note that this means diseases such as Dutch Elm Disease, killing 100 percent of American elm trees, and white nose syndrome which is killing 100 percent of bats. Fungi in humans cause things like ringworm and infectious dandruff, but they also cause several diseases most folks have not heard of such as histoplasmosis and coccidioidomycosis, which are essentially diseases we breathe in, and then they eat their way out in 1-2 percent of infected persons. Most of us instead develop what appears to be a serious cold. Thus, fungi do not kill humans very often, unless immune compromised.

I should note that women know a lot about fungi, as they develop *Candida* vaginal infections, which can be chronic and a "royal pain" for them. More recently, we see that *Candida* fungi are causing bloodstream infections in immune-compromised patients; for example, they are now the fourth leading cause, fourth to various bacteria. They are now becoming heavily studied because of the bloodstream infections. Why have they not been heavily studied as causing vaginal infections in women? The reason I think is because vaginal candidiasis, like menstrual toxic shock syndrome, is a women's disease. Until recently, women's health issues have always taken a back seat to other diseases. More grant dollars have gone to study Lyme Disease than either *Candida* infections or menstrual TSS. I remember Congress having to step in and mandate that the National Institutes of Health spend at least $1 billion per year on breast cancer research, since the National Institutes of Health and the scientific community could not make this happen on their own. Guess what? When grant dollars became available to study how to manage breast cancer, the fatality rate went down because new drugs were developed for use in treatment. I will mention one other case like this. As I said above, one person in seven, who dies worldwide, dies due to tuberculosis. Yes, that is correct, tuberculosis. I was sharing a taxi with a bacteriologist (Dr. Patrick Brennan) from Fort Collins, CO. At the time, he was the only researcher in the United States funded to study tuberculosis. When Congress found this out, they were horrified and mandated the funding of at least fifteen grants per year to study tuberculosis. It is clear to me that too often scientists on grant review panels cannot self-police, and this is how such distorted funding happens.

In other words, their area of research is always more interesting than causes of other diseases, and if they and their ilk populate grant review panels, distorted funding recommendations occur.

Parasite diseases are definitely the scourge of the world, but in the United States there are only a few that are common: 1) *Giardia* diarrhea; 2) *Trichomonas* sexually-transmitted infections; 3) toxoplasmosis; and 4) pinworms. At any given time, it is estimated that 15 percent of Americans have pinworms, diagnosed from intense butt-scratching associated with infection. Probably the most well-known parasitic infection is malaria, not common in the US but common worldwide, even as close as the Caribbean.

There are many microbes that do not cause disease, and indeed there are many that are helpful to us. They create yogurt, cheeses, bread, wine and beer, and degrade wastes. I will not go into these further since this book is about diseases.

On the opposing side of microbiology is immunology. The human immune system is designed to help us get rid of microbial pathogens (disease-causing agents), either through development of immunity, the result of infection, or through prior vaccination. The immune system is incredibly complex and internally redundant. Despite this complexity, most of us survive infections. Microbes have forever been at war with our immune systems, and indeed most microbes that cause disease trigger harmful inflammation, further promoting diseases. Microbes usually go through our mucous membranes to cause diseases, as opposed to skin, since mucous membranes are more permeable to disease agents than skin. Mucous membranes have other jobs, for example to allow food to gain access to the bloodstream through our intestines and for women to become pregnant. In the principal diseases talked about in this book, the causative bacteria make toxins that easily penetrate mucosal surfaces on their own to cause serious diseases.

There are two major subdivisions of your immune system. We call them innate (things you are born with) and adaptive (things that develop when you encounter foreign diseases). When you have a cut or scrape, within twenty-four hours, the site will become inflamed. This is because the major component of your innate immune system is also the major white blood cell type floating around inside you. We call them neutrophils or polymorphonuclear leukocytes (PMNs). PMNs make up 70 percent of your white blood cells, and they are easy to identify because they have a multi-lobed nucleus; why they have the lobed-appearance is not known. However, PMNs sense this cut or scrape and immediately enter the area to try to contain any infection that might occur. Their presence and immune activities typify inflammation. These cells are particularly good at getting rid of bacteria that normally live with you on your skin (we call the normal microbiome). Keep in mind that if you do not have a functioning immune system, those bacteria that are "normal" can kill you.

The second major part of your immune system is the adaptive immune system. It is a major target in toxic shock syndrome. This immune system is called "adaptive" since it takes about four days to kick into gear to help you fight off infections.

When I was seventeen years old and I was sitting in a study hall in high school, suddenly I developed shaking chills, a very high fever (104°F), and a violent cough. I had acquired a bacterial infection of the lungs called *Streptococcus pneumoniae* pneumonia. I was deathly sick for four days. I thought I was going to die. On day four, a miracle happened. My adaptive immune system finally kicked in, and I had produced antibodies to the causative bacteria. On day four, my fever "broke", meaning it came back to normal, my breathing got better, and I felt alive again. The cough remained as a delayed sequela for three months, but I lived.

There are two major components of the adaptive immune system, what we call humoral (meaning in the bloodstream) and cellular. The most important cells of the humoral immune system are white blood cells called B lymphocytes. These B lymphocytes produce antibodies about four days after exposure to foreign agents like *Streptococcus pneumoniae*. The antibodies are what made me get better on day four. They allowed the bacteria to be eliminated from me. B lymphocytes are also responsible for making antibodies against toxins (poisons) like TSS Toxin. By twelve years of age, 80 percent of humans will have antibodies against TSS Toxin and are resistant to the poisonous effects of the toxin. The diphtheria, whooping cough, tetanus, and polio vaccines all stimulate antibodies that neutralize the toxic effects of those toxins (poisons) or viruses. We vaccinate people to speed up the adaptive immune system. Vaccination allows the speed-up to be twenty-four hours instead of four days, so we do not ever develop disease. B lymphocytes make up about 10 percent of our white blood cells. It takes them four days to kick into gear because there are so few directed against any given foreign disease agent.

There may be one hundred thousand different things that B lymphocytes must respond to in order to protect us. With that great number of foreign things, there cannot be very many B lymphocytes of any specificity, and B lymphocytes are very specific for any given foreign agent. Put simply, it takes four days for the B lymphocytes to be in sufficient numbers to protect us. This may not seem optimal, and it is not, but here we are, still alive... so it does usually work.

There is another kind of lymphocyte, T lymphocytes. Their job is to help B lymphocytes and to kill difficult disease-causing agents like tuberculosis, fungal and parasite infections, and many viruses like measles, mumps, and rubella. T lymphocytes also take at least four days to kick into gear to help us fight off infections. Like B lymphocytes, they make up about 10 percent of white blood cells. They do not kill things by making antibodies. Instead, they either kill foreign things by activating other white blood cells, or they kill by making other kinds of toxic molecules. T lymphocytes are the major cells that are infected by HIV, leading to AIDS, and they are the major cells that become way over-activated to cause toxic shock syndrome (discussed a lot later).

There is one other major type of immune cell called macrophage meaning large cell that eats things. This cell type is activated by T lymphocytes primarily, and it comprises the remaining 10 percent of white blood cells. Macrophages have two major functions, namely to kill difficult bacteria like *Mycobacterium tuberculosis*, fungi, and protozoa, and to eat PMNs, mentioned above that have bacteria inside them. In other words, macrophages do not completely trust the ability of PMNs to kill microbes.

All of these immune processes are going on at the same time and for all kinds of microbes. I have just mentioned above some of the most important places where PMNs, B lymphocytes, T lymphocytes, and macrophages function. If you think about it, PMNs protect us against our own normal microbiome. B lymphocytes make antibodies to neutralize toxins and get rid of bacteria that live primarily outside of our cells. T lymphocytes kill virus-infected human cells and some difficult microbes. Macrophages are activated by T lymphocytes to kill all other disease-causing agents. And, with this immune system, we are protected from nearly everything, assuming we live the four days for our adaptive immune systems to kick in, assuming we have been vaccinated, or assuming some toxin like TSS Toxin is not causing immune dysfunction.

It is the interplay of innate and adaptive immune systems, with the greatest of complexity that is designed to keep us alive. Their jobs are to sense all the foreign things we encounter, including bacteria, viruses, fungi, protozoa, and other non-living, yet foreign, things found in dirt or dust. Although we know a lot about the immune system, we learn more each day of its remarkable complexity and abilities. As we learn more, the future becomes brighter that we will become better able to eliminate foreign disease-causing agents, prevent and treat autoimmunity, and treat cancers.

I perform research at the interface between how bacteria cause disease and how our immune systems protect us or are altered to dysfunctionality to make diseases more serious. These areas are called bacterial pathogenesis (genesis of pathology) and host defense. As noted previously, I received my first National Institutes of Health grant in 1979. I have been continually funded from then up to the present time, sometimes better-funded and sometimes worse. My research on pathogenesis and host defense will provide the major component of this book. My clinical colleagues and I have now described the causes of twenty-three new infectious diseases. This began with my publicizing a new disease in June of 1980 known as menstrual toxic shock syndrome. At that time as I said, I was in my first year as an Assistant Professor at the UCLA Medical Center in the Department of Microbiology and Immunology. The prior summer I had received a new grant, my first, from the National Institutes of Health, the National Institute of Allergy and Infectious Diseases, to study an infection with no name and which faculty members told me was not present in the Los Angeles area. I was told things like: "this must be a Midwestern disease", and "the disease cannot get across the mountains to Los Angeles." In fact, this disease, which as I said became known as menstrual TSS, was present across the United States and was present in other countries as we later found out. This book is a discussion of all aspects of toxic shock syndrome from my perspective, beginning at the beginning since I was there, and ending where we are today, with expectations for the future.

Toxic shock syndrome is a disease that actively requires participation of the human immune system. It is important for another reason: it is really the first time that the American public learned about the discovery process of an infectious disease, real time, affording them the opportunity to impact their own healthcare real time.

I consider this one of my most important service functions for the American public. Although some physicians and biomedical scientists objected to what I have done, I always think it is better for the public to be as informed as possible, particularly when their own healthcare is involved.

Chapter 6

Menstrual TOXIC SHOCK SYNDROME: The Beginning

You are now completely prepared to understand all aspects of toxic shock syndrome. Come along with me on the journey. I consider Louis Pasteur, the father of modern microbial pathogenesis and vaccination immunology, with wisdom when he said, "Chance favors only the prepared mind." This means that brilliance doesn't just happen, but instead it is the result of scientific preparation. I am no Louis Pasteur, but I think my mentors made me well prepared, or at least above average. Let me give you a quick example. Graduate students pursuing their doctorate degrees must each write research proposals in their second year, and they must defend them orally. There is a committee of five to six faculty members who evaluate the performance on this oral defense. One of my committee members, Dr. Al Markovetz, who I have mentioned previously, asked me to draw the structure of a Gram-negative bacterium. I asked him which one and into how much detail I should go. His response was: "Pick your favorite one, and then go into as much detail as you can." I knew a lot about the bacterium *Salmonella typhimurium*, the cause of millions of cases of severe diarrhea with high fever, down to the molecular level. So… that is what I started drawing on the chalkboard. After about thirty minutes, Al, seemingly stunned, said to me: "Pat, no one should know the structure of any bacterium in that much detail. You can stop now." My rationale for knowing the structure at the molecular level was that then I was prepared for anything related to Gram-negative bacteria in general, and that was true. You may ask what Gram-negative, as opposed to Gram-positive, which is the alternative is. Gram-negative bacteria have a weak wall around them, and when stained with a Safranin dye, they stain pink. Gram-positive bacteria have a strong cell wall around them, and when stained with Crystal Violet, they stain purple instead of pink. About half of disease-causing bacteria are Gram-negative, like *Salmonella, E. coli,* and *Yersinia pestis,* the latter being the cause of bubonic and pneumonic plagues. The alternatives are Gram-positive, and they include *Staphylococcus aureus, Streptococcus pyogenes,* and *Streptococcus pneumoniae. Mycobacterium tuberculosis* does not Gram-stain.

Toxic shock syndrome is the name given initially to a serious infection that was seen originally in a pediatric population, both males and females, without regard to menstrual status in the females. My friend Dr. James Todd, Denver Children's Hospital along with another friend of mine Dr. Frank Kapral from The Ohio State University published on the clinical features of toxic shock syndrome, gave it the name TSS, made the association with the bacterium *Staphylococcus aureus,* and proposed that "epidermolytic toxin" (a poison that separates the layers of the skin) was the cause.[16] This toxin later could not be associated with TSS, and it never has and in fact does not exist. Toxic shock syndrome was the name given to the disease because first the kids appeared "toxic", and thus some kind of toxin was the likely cause. Shock was added since the children developed a profound drop in blood pressure, which we know as shock. Shock literally means that the reduction in blood pressure is so profound that the organs are dying due to lack of oxygen. Despite the association with *Staphylococcus aureus,* Jim Todd called the infection a syndrome; this was unfortunate. Syndromes mean that we do not know the cause. Diseases mean we do know the cause. Thus, even though Jim and his colleagues called it a syndrome, it should have been called a disease since it was associated with *Staphylococcus aureus.* In a later chapter you will see why this naming as a syndrome was unfortunate. The Todd and Colleagues paper was published in a premier journal called *The Lancet* in the fall of 1978. The manuscript, although published in a strong journal, was largely ignored. Indeed, multiple publications came out previously and at about the same time describing the clinical disease correctly but giving it different names, such as "Adult Kawasaki Syndrome"[20] and "staphylococcal scarlet fever"[21]. Kawasaki Syndrome is typically seen in children under four years of age.[22,23] It has many overlapping clinical features with toxic shock syndrome, but even today there is no uniformly agreed upon cause of Kawasaki Syndrome. A physician, Dr. Christian Schrock in Minnesota, had also suggested that TSS is associated with herpes virus, and maybe herpes is the cause.[7] This combination of things is likely why Jim Todd did not call this a disease caused by *Staphylococcus aureus* but instead called it a syndrome. I have views on this that will be discussed later, but I want to return to the beginning.

Staphylococcal toxic shock syndrome is indeed the same as staphylococcal scarlet fever, occasionally described in the scientific literature, spanning the time across the 1900s. Jim Todd was unaware of those prior publications, going all the way back at least to 1919. I do not fault him for not knowing since he was primarily a clinician, but I would have thought the microbiologist Dr. Frank Kapral might have known. Also, at the time of the description, there was no internet, and it could be difficult to find access to old published papers. I knew of them only because as noted in a prior chapter, I was a postdoctoral associate in the world's expert laboratory on scarlet fever.

On my birthday (June 2, 1980), I spoke with a biomedical science writer from the *Los Angeles Times*. The writer, Harry Nelson (now deceased), wrote the story for the first Saturday of June (June 7) 1980. I had given him the symptoms patients would experience, the causative bacteria (*Staphylococcus aureus*), and the causative toxin (poison) that the bacteria were making that resulted in TSS. I ended our conversation with the following statement and advice: "Please have patients or their treating physicians notify the Los Angeles County Health Department to Report cases." Harry also called the CDC to add to my description and epidemiology of the disease. The story was exceptionally well written and presented. I think it is important for readers to remember that I was in my first year as a faculty member, an Assistant Professor in the Microbiology and Immunology Department at the University of California, Los Angeles (UCLA). I think it took a lot of guts to speak with the *Los Angeles Times* writer since this would affect the entire United States Healthcare System. Early on I was indeed criticized by some MD (physician) scientists and PhD scientists. However, I had tried for two years to convince the scientific and medical communities that there was in fact a disease, and these attempts were completely unsuccessful. When asked, I stated many times that my only loyalty was to the American public instead of the biomedical community since the American public was paying taxes that went to support my grant funding from the National Institutes of Health. Do I regret doing this? Emphatically... no!

I should address this point about trying to convince researchers and clinicians of this new disease a bit more thoroughly by making a few more points. While I was doing postdoctoral training at the University of Minnesota (1976-1979) studying the scarlet fever toxins, faculty colleagues came to me with teenage daughters of their friends, where the daughters had an exceptionally serious disease that looked exactly like serious scarlet fever. However, the bacteria that caused scarlet fever, *Streptococcus pyogenes*, were not present in the daughters. How could this have been? I was asked to help in figuring out what was going on since the laboratory in which I was working was indeed the premier laboratory in the world studying scarlet fever.

Scarlet fever is caused by the bacteria *Streptococcus pyogenes* (a.k.a. Group A streptococci). These bacteria are the causes of "strep throat", wherein about ten million United States children per year develop strep throat. It is noteworthy that Group A streptococcal infections are easily treated with penicillin antibiotics. This bacterium has always remained susceptible to antibiotics, an interesting and yet unexplained phenomenon, since other bacteria relatively easily develop resistance. For example, *Staphylococcus aureus* very easily develops resistance to antibiotics. Today, nearly 50 percent of *Staphylococcus aureus* bacteria in hospitals are highly resistant to all penicillin and cephalosporin antibiotics; we know them as methicillin-resistant *Staphylococcus aureus* (MRSA). Additionally, 100 percent of *Staphylococcus aureus* in the United States are resistant to the most basic penicillin antibiotics (penicillin G, penicillin VK, and ampicillin). In contrast 100 percent of Group A streptococci are susceptible to penicillin antibiotics. Today, Group A streptococcal infections are routinely treated with another antibiotic called azithromycin since this requires only three days of treatment instead of ten days for penicillin antibiotics.

Although Group A streptococci are the cause of pharyngitis (strep throat), some varieties of the microbe also cause scarlet fever. There are more than one hundred kinds of Group A streptococci in the United States. Thus, it is possible to develop strep throat multiple times; immunity Group A strep depends on specific antibodies to each of the one hundred varieties. For an unknown reason, adults have a higher intrinsic resistance to Group A streptococcal infection. Thus, when we think of strep throat, we think of kids.

Back in the early 1900s, Group A streptococcal infections often resulted in a particularly serious disease called malignant scarlet fever . Indeed, there were special wings of hospitals for these patients to keep them away from others to prevent disease spread. This malignant scarlet fever resulted in the deaths of many children, and occasionally adults. If you have read children's books by Beatrix Potter, of Peter Rabbit fame, you will know that the book *The Velveteen Rabbit* by Margery Williams describes a stuffed rabbit that comes to life.[24] The story also describes a boy who developed scarlet fever where all the toys, including stuffed animals, had to be burned to prevent infection spread. The real point is that scarlet fever could have been highly fatal at that time.

It should also be noted that in the early 1900s, there were no penicillin antibiotics to treat these infections; penicillin only became available at the time of World War II. For an unknown reason, the serious scarlet fever of the early 1900s disappeared in the 1950s to become what many physicians called scarlatina, a very mild version of the same serious scarlet fever. This is important to discuss since many recent physicians were trained only to think that scarlet fever was mild and not particularly a serious problem in the 1980s.

In my studies, I have come to appreciate that Group A streptococcal strains cycle in populations, like in the United States, in roughly thirty-five-year intervals, likely dependent on overall immunity in the population. We call this herd immunity. When the majority of the human population is immune, the bacteria can no longer spread, because of rarity of transmission to non-immune people. This happened with Group A streptococci in the 1950s, but in the 1980s, the serious form of scarlet fever reappeared (discussed later), likely because of lack of residual immune persons in the overall human population. It caught the medical community by surprise since they had been taught scarlet fever was now mild, causing only the scarlatina.

It is also noteworthy that some physicians began not even treating strep throat with antibiotics. Do you know just how bad this is... not treating with antibiotics? I have already stated that there is little antibiotic resistance in Group A streptococci, so treating streptococcal infections should not be viewed as overuse of antibiotics. However, the reason strep throat is treated ALWAYS with antibiotics is because not treating can result in what we call a delayed sequela. In other word, there can be a sequel disease called rheumatic fever. Rheumatic fever is defined by arthritis, heart damage, usually seen as mitral valve scarring, and a shaking neurological disease called Syndenham's chorea (Saint Vitus Dance). Rheumatic fever is a "forever" life-changing experience and is easily prevented, as shown by one of my mentors and colleagues Dr. Lewis Wannamaker (now deceased) by treating infections with penicillin.

As noted above, I was asked to help figure out why daughters of friends were developing serious scarlet fever, but Group A streptococci were not isolated. In 1978-1979 alone, I was asked to help in twenty-two cases. A highly unique feature of scarlet fever is the presence of a sunburn-like rash and thus, the term "scarlet" in the name. Notice I said daughters in all cases. Each of these daughters had this sunburn-like rash. Additionally, scarlet fever is also defined by the term "fever". The toxins (poisons) produced by Group A streptococci, related to TSS Toxin, are the most potent fever-causing agents (a.k.a. pyrogens) known. Fever in people results from the toxic effects of the toxins on the hypothalamus part of the brain. In the later 1970s, Dennis Watson and I worked out the pathway of these toxins leading to fever.[25] We showed that the toxins acted on the hypothalamus part of the brain to cause the release of molecules called prostaglandins, notably prostaglandin E2. Aspirin and related molecules block the production of prostaglandins, and that is why they can reduce fever. After prostaglandin production, fever results from altering a normal set point of 98.6°F though altering the ratio in the brain of two other molecules, the "feel good" molecule serotonin, and the "melancholy" molecule norepinephrine. When the ratio of these two molecules is altered, nerves are affected that cause the person to shiver, feel cold and put on a sweater, and increase metabolism to generate body heat. The pathway to fever becomes pretty easy to understand.

In its severest form, as present in the early 1900s, a dramatic drop in blood pressure can be seen in malignant scarlet fever patients. These daughters also had this dramatic drop in blood pressure; we call it hypotension. This means that the liquid part of blood is leaking into body tissues, rather than remaining in the blood vessels, a condition we call capillary leak. When the liquid part of blood leaks into tissues, overall blood flow in the body is reduced, and the body organs cannot receive sufficient oxygen to keep them alive. If this is serious enough, the organs will stop functioning, leading to what we call shock, as in toxic "shock" syndrome, and death can result soon thereafter. One of the first organs to be affected and shut down is the kidneys. The kidneys are the only way the toxins can be removed from the patient, so having kidney shut-down allows the toxin to continue causing serious disease.

Scarlet fever is caused by Group A streptococcal strains (or types) that make particular toxins (poisons) that the bacteria secrete into their surrounding environment. These scarlet fever toxins as I said are the most potent pyrogens known, they cause a sunburn-like rash, and they cause the blood vessels to leak. This is the reason scarlet fever of the early 1900s was so serious. There are two major scarlet fever toxins, called streptococcal scarlet fever toxins (or streptococcal pyrogenic exotoxins) A and C. Scarlet fever toxin A was the toxin that caused nearly all cases of malignant scarlet fever in the early 1900s. I have a large number of Group A streptococci from such patients, preserved since then as freeze-dried bacteria, and they all produce scarlet fever toxin A. Immunity in the United States population resulted in the disappearance of the malignant scarlet fever for thirty-five years, only to reemerge in the 1980s. Also, in the early 1900s, there were attempts to develop vaccines against scarlet fever toxin A, just like what was done for diphtheria and tetanus, two other toxin diseases where in fact we have terrific vaccines today. When diphtheria was common, companies also prepared antibodies to diphtheria toxin in horses. This antibody could be given to non-vaccinated persons with diphtheria to neutralize the potent diphtheria toxin that if left untreated would kill the person by stopping the heart. At the same time, like malignant scarlet fever, there were separate wings of hospitals to isolate diphtheria patients from others to prevent spread. I have a large bottle of "Lederle" horse antibody against scarlet fever toxin A that was used to help treat scarlet fever patients in the early 1900s. It should be noted that scarlet fever toxin A was purified to relative homogeneity by Drs. George and Gladys Dick in 1926 . I also have some of their purified toxin in my laboratory, as well as antibodies to the toxin as raised in rabbits. Thus, I know with certainty that their toxin was the same as we see today. Lederle later changed its name to Lederle-Praxis, and still later to other names. The important thing to remember is that this company was instrumental in developing many of the vaccines we use today, for example the Hib vaccine that all children receive to prevent a serious, life-threatening form of meningitis and serious, life-threatening "sticky throat" infection (blocking the ability to breathe, called epiglottitis).

Now, you see why these colleagues with teens with malignant scarlet fever were coming to me. I became a world expert on scarlet fever as caused by Group A streptococci. As also stated above, Group A streptococci were not isolated from the teens. Thus, there had to be a different cause. I also knew that there was a bacterium related to Group A streptococci; this bacterium has already been mentioned many times... *Staphylococcus aureus*. I noticed that in 100 percent of the twenty-two cases in the teens, *Staphylococcus aureus* was always present in cultures from the throat and other body sites, including the vagina. Thus, I thought that *Staphylococcus aureus* was likely causing the disease.

You could ask: "Pat, why did you think so?" My response is that the kids could die of their infections, so we lose nothing in thinking that the "related" bacterium *Staphylococcus aureus* was the likely cause. Many if not all of these teens were indeed treated with broad-acting (we call broad-spectrum) antibiotics to even cover for *Staphylococcus aureus* infection.

It is now important to keep in mind that this disease looked like malignant scarlet fever, and so I thought the disease was caused by a related scarlet fever-like toxin produced by *Staphylococcus aureus*. This turned out to be true, with my isolation of the causative toxin called TSS Toxin. Physicians can treat infections with antibiotics, but the toxin produced by the causative bacteria will continue to have its effects since the toxin is not alive and cannot be killed by antibiotics; it is a protein more than ten thousand times smaller than the bacteria. This is the reason Lederle was making horse antibodies against scarlet fever toxin A—that is, to treat patients with Group A streptococcal scarlet fever.

Horse antibodies neutralize the scarlet fever toxin A by inactivating its toxicity. At that time, the daughters of friends were not treated with intravenous antibodies since it was not known and not agreed upon that a toxin, much less the bacteria *Staphylococcus aureus*, was the cause.

In looking back, there are several important things about these daughters that were important in later studies. They were all teenage girls. They were all using tampons during their menstrual periods. They all had a serious scarlet fever-like disease with accompanying high fever and drop in blood pressure (hypotension) during their menstrual periods. This dramatic drop in blood pressure resulted in shut-down first of the kidneys. I reasoned that if this is indeed a toxin-mediated disease, the kidney shut down would allow more of the toxin to remain in the bloodstream to cause even more serious disease.

It quickly became standard of care for physicians to treat patients with this new disease with fluid and electrolytes to keep blood pressure as normal as possible. This would allow the causative toxin to be eliminated. Through the kidneys is indeed the only way the causative toxin can be removed from the body. In a study I performed in a rabbit model of this disease, I used radioactive toxin to follow it in the body. The toxin accumulates the most in the kidneys and the T lymphocytes of the adaptive immune system. The kidney damage seen in this disease is almost certainly because of toxin accumulation. I knew at that time (1978) that the effect on the immune system was the most important activity leading to blood vessel leak and thus, serious disease. What was happening to the teenage girls was that a toxin (TSS Toxin) was tremendously over-activating their immune systems, causing release of soluble factors from immune cells that were then causing fever, hypotension, and scarlet fever-like or sunburn-like rash. Through lots of subsequent research, we now know that all of this is true.

Back in June 1980, I came into my office on the following Monday morning (June 9, 1980) after the Saturday publicity to find more than one hundred news reporters in the hall, waiting to speak with me about TSS. I had no idea how quickly this had spread, even including CBS national news. In the next six months I literally spoke with thousands of reporters, such that menstrual TSS became the second-greatest news event of 1980, second only to the Iran Hostage Crisis, which had gone on the entire year instead of half a year. The result was that the American public learned about the disease concurrent with the biomedical community.

The CDC will say, and they have said many times, that they started the publicity on menstrual toxic shock syndrome. That is simply not the case. Although they had a "Morbidity and Mortality Weekly Report" publication on toxic shock syndrome, the Harry Nelson article in the *Los Angeles Times*, with follow-up reporting by the news media nationally, was the pivotal story that made menstrual TSS a household name.

For the next several months, the news on toxic shock syndrome exploded. I was so bombarded by answering news media questions that I cannot remember all of them. However, I responded to 100 percent of news media requests for information. I felt it was my job. I do remember some memorable interviews. I will give a few examples.

A reporter for the *Kansas City Star* newspaper asked me: "Is there somebody a little older I can speak to about this disease?"

I replied: "Nope just me." We had a great discussion of TSS and its cause.

I remember Midwest reporters calling my home at 4:00 A.M. in Los Angeles to speak with me (6:00 A.M. Midwest time), not remembering there was a two-hour time difference between the Midwest and Los Angeles. For many of these interviews, I followed the livestock report in the early morning. Through all of this, I did the interviews with as much enthusiasm as I could muster.

I also remember receiving a phone call from a woman from the Los Angeles County Health Department, Dr. Shirley Fannin, noting the very large number of calls they were receiving, and at the same time the disease association with the highest absorbency tampons. As huge media attention was paid to the disease, it quickly became clear that the CDC was blaming the Rely® tampons, made by Procter & Gamble, for the disease. I will get into a long discussion later of why this was so wrong, but for the moment let me say that Shirley Fannin and I noted that the risk of menstrual TSS depended primarily on the tampon absorbency, not the brand of tampon. In other words, Los Angeles was seeing cases associated with Rely®, but also Tampax®, Kotex®, and Playtex® of the highest absorbencies. We also noticed the exclusive association of menstrual TSS with *Staphylococcus aureus* bacteria.

During the first week of the news media spectacle on menstrual toxic shock syndrome and its high association with use of high-absorbency tampons, I met with Dr. Jim Widder of Procter & Gamble. He was my first company contact of any tampon manufacturer. This company produced and sold the Rely® tampons, tampons highly associated with menstrual TSS. Jim and I met for lunch at a restaurant owned by Sonny Bono (of Sonny and Cher fame and now deceased) in Westwood, just South of the UCLA campus. Jim asked me where I thought this menstrual TSS "process" was likely to go. Here is what I told Jim.

The disease is caused by *Staphylococcus aureus*. It turns out, unknown to me, that another friend of mine Dr. Christian Shrock from Minnesota had found a disease with the acronym SAD MADAME that turned out to be menstrual TSS. Dr. Shrock thought the disease might be caused by herpes virus, as he published in the scientific literature.[7] Because of the significant alteration of immune system function in menstrual TSS, patients latently infected with herpes virus will have their herpes pop out of latency and cause overt infections. Toxic shock syndrome is not caused by herpes. At this time, the CDC would not say that menstrual TSS was caused by *Staphylococcus aureus*. They were clearly ignoring the work of Jim Todd's and my group of researchers.

The CDC researchers were not the only skeptics. I used to play racquetball with a graduate student at UCLA. He commented to me multiple times in later years that he did not do research as a graduate student in my laboratory, because he "just could not see how this disease and tampon association could be real". He did fine in another laboratory and is a well-regarded researcher at a major public university.

I also told Jim Widder that the disease is not a syndrome with unknown cause but instead, is a form of scarlet fever but now caused by a scarlet fever toxin produced by *Staphylococcus aureus*. I explained to Jim how the toxin causes fever, where the reduction in blood pressure comes from, and why we see the scarlet fever-like rash, all the result of bad effects on the human immune system.

I then explained that many tampons, mostly those of highest absorbency were associated with menstrual TSS. I noted that it is important to define what we mean by menstrual TSS. Menstrual means only that the disease is occurring during the roughly seven-day timeframe when women are menstruating. It does not say anything about where the *Staphylococcus aureus* bacteria will be found in the patients.

Thus, as I mentioned previously, in the twenty-two young women with this new disease with which I was helping out, the bacteria *Staphylococcus aureus* were isolated from multiple mucous membranes, including the throat and vagina. Thus, I told Jim it was important to say: "menstrual, vaginal TSS" when the disease was associated with vaginal presence of *Staphylococcus aureus* during menstruation.

I have said much about Group A streptococci and scarlet fever. I have tried multiple times, unsuccessfully, to publish that streptococcal scarlet fever occurs most often in young and older women of menstrual age, during their menstrual periods. I guess the scientific community does not want to know this. However, it is true, and it has a strong bearing later in lawsuits against tampon manufacturers as I will discuss in a separate chapter. For now, it is only important to know that I told Jim Widder about streptococcal scarlet fever and how it occurs.

I told Jim that he and Procter & Gamble should be prepared for lots of legal issues with Rely® tampons, but TSS also occurs in males and females not associated with tampons. Thus, tampons are not the direct cause of TSS but *Staphylococcus aureus* is. Tampons have a co-causal role. Jim asked why I thought tampons were associated with menstrual TSS, and specifically why Rely® brand was associated. I told Jim: "Rely® is only one of many associated tampons. However, Procter & Gamble Rely® is the 'new kid' on the block, and this is the reason there is so much focus on that specific tampon. Other high-absorbency tampons also are associated with menstrual TSS." So, why did I say new kid on the block? Procter & Gamble began marketing Rely® tampons in 1980, going from no sales to having 25 percent of the tampon market share by the summer of 1980. If any of you know Procter & Gamble, you will know of their magnificent ability to market products. Think of Tide®, Pampers®, Crest®, and Head and Shoulders®. It turns out that Procter & Gamble had sent free samples of Rely® tampons through the mail to nearly all women in the United States. Procter & Gamble also has the thinking to improve on design of products when those products enter the market. Thus, Rely® tampons looked different from other tampons. Rely® tampons looked like tea bags filled with white chips and foam pieces in the bags. All other tampons look like compressed cotton and rayon in a relatively tubular form. The white chips in the Rely® tampons were a form of a chemical called carboxy-methyl cellulose (their form was called cross-linked derivative) whose purpose was to absorb menstrual blood, which they did well.

One other key point on this topic is that a member of the CDC task force on this new disease, menstrual TSS, in the San Francisco area stood next to a display of Rely® tampons, and said on national television: "If you've had this disease, notify the CDC." I hope you can see why the CDC came to emphasize the association with Rely®. Many women with menstrual TSS associated with Rely® tampons actually reported their cases to the CDC. However, many women, who developed menstrual TSS, and when they were using other tampons, did not report their cases to the CDC. It is interesting that a study was subsequently done which showed that women who developed menstrual TSS in association with non-Rely® tampon brands would later change their stated tampon use to Rely®. Few, if any women changed their minds in the opposite direction. Thus, it is clear that the major reason for the initial CDC focus on Rely® instead of all high-absorbency tampons occurred to a large extent because of this initial CBS news report from San Francisco. In other words, there was a strong news media bias.

Jim asked about the toxin that causes menstrual, vaginal TSS. I told him it was a scarlet fever-like toxin. Later I showed this scarlet fever-like toxin was a brand-new toxin called TSS Toxin.

I told Jim that rabbits, but not mice, could be used to study TSS. A lot of researchers use mice today to study human diseases, but this cannot be done with TSS.[12] Although not done yet at the time I spoke with Jim, seventeen humans have now purposely been injected with one or another of the TSS toxins, and all developed symptoms of TSS. Some almost died from their TSS. Some required admission to intensive care units in hospitals for up to two weeks. You may then ask the obvious question: "Who needs an animal model when we have seventeen humans who have been injected and developed disease." Perhaps you can ask: "What were they thinking?"

Another aside is important here. I attended a scientific meeting where a research presenter stated that the only virulence factor produced by Group A streptococci was the M protein on the surface of the bacteria. He went on to describe the activities of the M protein in the greatest of detail. After his presentation, there was a question and answer period, where I asked the first question. I asked: "How about you inject me with a small amount of M protein, and I inject you with a small amount of scarlet fever toxin A, and we will see if M protein is the only important virulence factor?" He of course backtracked and said that M protein would not be toxic, but the scarlet fever toxin A may kill him.

He said: "I meant the only important bacterial cell-surface virulence factor." I bring this up for one reason only. For some unknown and long-standing reason, the research community has never wanted these scarlet fever-like toxins to be important in human diseases. If I had to guess the reason, it is because the researchers studying them are in the Midwest and West, and at public universities, so they could not possibly be important.

I could not tell Jim Widder why tampons were associated with menstrual, vaginal TSS, except to say that Rely® was not the only associated tampon, so the composition was not important. Remember, Procter & Gamble made their Rely® tampon different from other tampons. I stated, therefore, that tampons were introducing something from the outside, not intrinsic within the tampons. We now know from my 1983 publication in the *Journal of Infectious Diseases* that the something introduced was air (oxygen), required for *Staphylococcus aureus* to produce the toxin.[15]

At a later date, Jim Widder told me that what I told him during our meeting in June of 1980 came true.

Very soon after my meeting with Jim Widder, Procter & Gamble called together what they referred to as an external Scientific Advisory Group (SAG) meeting in Cincinnati where Procter & Gamble is based. I remember most of the external committee in addition to me: Drs. Michael Osterholm (Minnesota State Epidemiologist), Jeffrey Davis (Wisconsin State Epidemiologist), Jim Todd (Denver Pediatrician who gave the name toxic shock syndrome to TSS), and for some unknown reason Brain MacMahon (now deceased but former cancer epidemiologist from Harvard University). Brian was a serious problem at the meeting to say the least. He had just published an epidemiology paper showing coffee was associated with cancer. The coffee brand, Folgers® was marketed by Procter & Gamble, so it appeared to me Brian came in with a "chip on his shoulder", knowing ahead of time that Rely® tampons, also marketed by Procter & Gamble, were the only problem in menstrual, vaginal TSS. I thought this meeting was a complete waste of time. Later epidemiology studies showed that coffee was NOT associated with increased risk of cancer, and all high-absorbency tampons, not just Rely®, were associated with menstrual TSS.

What Was I Thinking? Toxic Shock Syndrome

For all of June and July, I addressed news media regularly. At the same time, the CDC had set up a TSS Task Force. This was overseen by Dr. John Bennett. However, EIS officers were appointed as direct heads. EIS means Epidemic Intelligence Service officers or "disease detectives" in CDC common language. The chief of the TSS task force was Dr. Kathryn Shands. Dr. Bruce Dan (now deceased) was the deputy chief of the task force. I interacted regularly with these two CDC folks. I found Kathryn to be a likeable person with a "good head". In contrast, Bruce unfortunately at the time could be a real problem—that is, the "bad cop" in a good cop-bad cop scenario, with Kathryn being the good cop. I will be giving examples along the way in this book of what I mean. Bruce and I became friends later after he left the CDC and became an editor of the *Journal of the American Medical Association* or as most of us know it *JAMA*. Later he did a show in New York called *Ask Doctor Dan*.

Since I had started the major publicity, the TSS Task Force was forced to interact with me. The first thing they asked was why I thought *Staphylococcus aureus* was the cause, and furthermore, why did I think a new toxin was the proximal (immediate) cause? I explained about the twenty-two cases I had participated in while in Minnesota and how 100 percent of these teenage young women using tampons had developed the disease in association with *Staphylococcus aureus* and a new toxin. I remember the TSS Task Force asked: "How could you rule out herpes virus as the cause?" I explained that the toxin was altering immune system function, causing immune dysfunction, and this allowed herpes to pop out of its latent state in the chromosomes of patients, and only coincidentally to be associated with the disease.

The TSS task force then challenged me to prove I was correct. They asked: "What do you need from us to satisfy your thinking that *Staphylococcus aureus* is the cause, and to be able to tell us what toxin was the proximal cause of TSS?" I asked them to isolate *Staphylococcus aureus* from the vaginas of young women with menstrual TSS and at the same time isolate *Staphylococcus aureus* from a roughly equal number of matched, young women who did not have menstrual TSS, the latter group what we call controls. I told them that these isolates should be sent to me in what is called blinded conditions. Blinded means the *Staphylococcus aureus* isolates from patients and controls were randomly assigned numbers from 1-60. I was supposed to identify those that came from menstrual, vaginal toxic shock syndrome, and which ones were from controls.

The CDC TSS task force did in fact send me the blinded isolates, numbered 1-60. This was in July 1980. The first thing this said to me was that the CDC could isolate *Staphylococcus aureus* vaginally from women. It turns out that nearly 100 percent of the menstrual TSS patients from their collection had *Staphylococcus aureus* vaginally, whereas only about one-third of the controls were positive for *Staphylococcus aureus* vaginally. Thus, these studies alone showed a high association of menstrual, vaginal TSS with *Staphylococcus aureus*, thus fulfilling two of Koch's postulates.

Now, remember that I said earlier that are many strains of *Staphylococcus aureus*. If *Staphylococcus aureus* is the cause, then the question now is could I now find the one unique toxin (poison) that is causing the menstrual TSS? Imagine for a minute how difficult this task was. *Staphylococcus aureus* in general makes three thousand proteins based on the number of genes in its chromosome. By the way, gene sequencing was not available in 1980, so we did not really know at the time how many proteins *Staphylococcus aureus* could make. I had to find the "one". Many of these proteins would be expected to be shared among strains, but there are some expected differences among strains, for example in kinds of toxins (poisons) that might be produced. Could I find the one toxin out of three thousand proteins that was specific for the menstrual TSS women and not the controls? I had to develop a way to identify that one unique toxin associated with cases but not controls.

Here was my thinking and what I did. First, I knew the toxin had to be a scarlet fever-like toxin. These toxins are secreted by the bacteria into humans as the *Staphylococcus aureus* become late in their growth, using up easily available food, a phase of growth we call post-exponential phase of growth. This means when food becomes short, the bacteria become threatened, and they then make toxins (poisons) to disable humans and particularly their immune systems. This in turn allows them to spread out and find more food. Remember, I said previously that human *Staphylococcus aureus* must overwhelm the human immune system to survive. To do this, they express genes for production of toxins that attack the immune system, doing what we call dysregulation; in other words the *Staphylococcus aureus* bacteria "screw-up" our immune systems. This allows them to survive and spread.

I often ask folks who is smarter, *Staphylococcus aureus* or humans? Nearly all say humans are smarter. Humans obviously have brains, and *Staphylococcus aureus* does not. However, what intrinsic right do we as humans have to define brain by this blob of stuff in our heads, or its surrogate intelligence? *Staphylococcus aureus* does not have a brain as we think about brains. However, they win the numbers game in that they outnumber us tremendously in nearly any environment. For example, there are ten trillion *Staphylococcus aureus* bacteria in one cubic inch. Think of it this way, some humans, colonized by *Staphylococcus aureus*, have the equivalent of one-fourth of a stick of margarine on their skin, or the ten trillion I mention above.[26] I chose margarine to represent *Staphylococcus aureus* because it is gold in color like colonies of *Staphylococcus aureus*. Imagine smearing one-fourth of a stick of margarine all over your body. Now imagine doing the same thing in the noses, throats, eyes, and vaginas of women. This would define how many *Staphylococcus aureus* bacteria women have, who develop menstrual TSS. It is also well known that about one bacterium in ten million is a mutant. These mutations mean that the accumulated population of *Staphylococcus aureus* have millions of mutants that can adapt to nearly any human environment. Kind of like having a brain, possibly even better than having the human brain.

Now, let's return to my goal that summer of 1980, namely finding the one toxin in a haystack of three thousand proteins. Also, remember that hundreds of microbiologists over the years did not find the toxin, going back even to the father of modern immunology, Nobel Laureate Sir Frank Macfarlane Burnet, who identified a toxin he called alpha toxin in 1928.[27] Alpha toxin is a poison that kills red blood cells and immune cells that find themselves adjacent to *Staphylococcus aureus*. The toxin does not act systemically in the body to kill immune cells but only functions locally at the site of infections. I knew this toxin, alpha toxin, could NOT be the toxin I was looking for. Alpha toxin is mostly not produced by *Staphylococcus aureus* growing on human mucous membranes. The reason for this is that the toxin is required for production of boils on the skin and thus, is important for skin infections, but it is too toxic locally to be found on mucous membranes. If too much alpha toxin was produced on mucosal surfaces, the mucosa would be degraded, and the *Staphylococcus aureus* would easily spread into the bloodstream. Young women with menstrual, vaginal TSS typically do not have TSS *Staphylococcus aureus* in the bloodstream.

Dr. Patrick M. Schlievert

I knew the toxin I was searching for had to be a scarlet fever-like toxin like I said, and I also knew that the scarlet fever-like toxins are virtually indestructible, even in the face of complete exposure to 80 percent alcohol, a concentration that would kill any human or animal, and would even destroy nearly all of the three thousand proteins that can be produced by *Staphylococcus aureus*. I do not mean just drinking a small amount of 160 proof alcohol. Instead, I mean complete immersion in amounts that add up to 160 proof or 80 percent final concentration. I thus grew the sixty strains from the CDC in excellent growth media that favored toxin production, to stationary phase of growth (just past post-exponential phase) when toxins should be produced. I then treated the cultures with alcohol to achieve 80 percent final concentration. Maybe I should have drunk the alcohol instead to calm my nerves! However, the 80 percent alcohol killed the staphylococcal bacteria and destroyed all but a few of the three thousand proteins. It left three to five proteins intact, including scarlet fever-like toxins. I developed a way to separate these three to five proteins so I could look at them one at a time. I found one protein that I called pyrogenic (fever-producing) exotoxin (secreted toxin) type C (staphylococcal PE C) which was produced by one-half of the isolates and not produced by the other one-half. I identified two other scarlet fever-like toxins, designated staphylococcal PE A and PE B. I knew that staphylococcal PE A was produced by many of the isolates, and staphylococcal PE B was produced by only a few. It turned out that staphylococcal PE A was an already described toxin called staphylococcal enterotoxin A. As later data showed, this toxin (PE A) is indeed produced by 80 percent of menstrual TSS isolates, but it is produced in such low amounts, it cannot cause menstrual, vaginal TSS. Staphylococcal PE B turned out also to be another known staphylococcal toxin, in reality two toxins called staphylococcal enterotoxins B and C. These two highly related toxins, we know today, cause 50 percent of non-menstrual TSS. These two toxins (poisons) are produced in very high concentrations, just as I showed the staphylococcal PE C was produced in very high concentrations. However, these two toxins are produced by only 15 percent of menstrual, vaginal TSS isolates. When I grow menstrual TSS *Staphylococcus aureus* strain called MN8, from the eighth patient identified in Minnesota in 1980, in good culture media, this bacterial strain will produce thirty thousand micrograms of staphylococcal PE C (now called TSS Toxin) in each teaspoon of media. Consider that it requires only a tenth of a microgram per human to cause menstrual TSS (if the toxin is given directly into the bloodstream). That means I can easily produce enough of this toxin in one teaspoon to cause TSS in three hundred thousand persons if the toxin is given into the bloodstream. Today, as I produce this toxin, I culture the MN8 bacteria in one thousand teaspoons of media, the equivalent of an amount to cause TSS in three hundred million persons if the toxin gains access to the bloodstream. Practically speaking, this toxin (poison) that we know today as TSS Toxin can easily be produced in very high amounts.

Let's go back now to the blinded study I was doing. While I was developing the method to isolate the *Staphylococcus aureus* three to five proteins, and doing the exact same tests on all sixty coded isolates, Dr. Bruce Dan from the CDC called me every-other-day to "pick on" me. He believed I could not find the one toxin causing menstrual TSS. In this way, he could greatly strengthen the challenge to me to find the correct isolates.

I also remember me calling the TSS task force one day during this time to ask a question about menstrual TSS, noting that the CDC is supposed to work for all of us as Americans. I asked them if the CDC menstrual TSS task force had noticed that TSS patients also had developed an autoimmune disease called immune thrombocytopenic purpura, where the patients' own immune systems were destroying their platelets. If the patients indeed had this disease, they would forever have had their platelets destroyed by the immune system. One way to manage the disease is to remove the spleens which then reduces the amounts of antibodies produced that attack and destroy platelets. This was routinely done for such patients at that time. The problem is that the patients become susceptible to bloodstream infections later in life since they lack their spleens and thus, lack antibodies to fight off infections.

The task force would not give me an answer to the question, but they told me they knew the answer. In other words, they refused to tell me if menstrual TSS patients had immune thrombocytopenic purpura as a component of their toxic shock syndrome. Because the CDC TSS task force would not tell me the answer, some menstrual TSS patients had their spleens removed as a precaution against immune thrombocytopenic purpura. It turns out that even though the immune system does attack platelets in menstrual TSS patients, leading to very low platelet numbers and the possibility of a bleeding disorder, this is only transient in TSS patients, and goes away when the disease goes away. Thus, these patients did not need their spleens removed. This led me to submit a short manuscript to the *New England Journal of Medicine* asking the question of whether menstrual TSS patients have concurrent autoimmune diseases. I have already mentioned some overlapping autoimmune diseases earlier in this book. My submitted manuscript was never published, and I mean even today it remains unpublished. I should also note that many patients with menstrual TSS can be confused with having systemic lupus erythematosus, and the reverse is also true, due to overlapping symptoms. Many patients also have abnormal antibodies against their own DNA, a marker for systemic lupus erythematosus. These antibodies go away upon recovery from TSS, but they do not go away in bona fide systemic lupus erythematosus.

I will never forget this conversation, because it turned into a shouting match. I said, how dare they jeopardize the American public by not giving me the answer, which they knew. I did remind them that they works on behalf of the American public; they just laughed at me. They also said that the CDC was going to publish a paper on this, and I would just have to wait for it to be published. Such a paper was never published, so this remains an issue even today: Why do platelet numbers drop so dramatically? I would ask: "What were they thinking?"

In late July or early August of 1980, I called Kathryn Shands, chief of the CDC TSS task force, and I informed her that I was ready to unblind the samples. In other words, I thought I could correctly identify the toxic shock syndrome and non-toxic shock syndrome *Staphylococcus aureus* strains. I decided to go with what I called staphylococcal pyrogenic exotoxin C (PE C) as the likely causative toxin, both because of its 50:50 split (yes and no) and its high concentration of being produced. Kathryn came to my laboratory (and office) at UCLA, and later that morning Bruce Dan came. Bruce arrived about an hour after the samples became unblinded. I knew from his immediate hyperactivity that he was itching to laugh at me for incorrect identification. It turned out that Kathryn also did not believe I would be able to identify the isolates, so she did not even bring the unblinded code along with her. She had to call the other members of the TSS task force at the CDC in Atlanta to unblind the isolates. I had given her the list of which numbers I thought were from TSS patients, based on PE C production, and which were not from TSS patients, based on not producing this toxin (poison).

Quickly during her call from my office to the CDC, I could tell that she was absolutely stunned. She gasped and even turned white sitting across from me. I had in fact correctly identified the *Staphylococcus aureus* strains from menstrual TSS patients, and then by difference I had identified those not from menstrual, vaginal toxic shock syndrome. I also noted that the toxic shock syndrome strains did not produce the toxin, alpha toxin, whereas the non-toxic shock syndrome isolates had the ability to produce small amounts.

I re-mention alpha toxin here, because a friend of mine Dr. Roger Stone (he will be mentioned again in this book as one of the "good" guys) told me a couple years later that he had developed a way to visualize nearly all three thousand *Staphylococcus aureus* proteins. There were only two differences from his studies of menstrual TSS isolates and non-toxic shock syndrome isolates. TSS isolates produced the toxin I identified, pyrogenic exotoxin C (which in 1984 became known as TSS Toxin as discussed later in this book), but they did not produce much, if any alpha toxin. In contrast, non-toxic shock syndrome isolates did not produce PE C and did produce alpha toxin.

I should also add that I had purified PE C to purity as determined biochemically. I showed that the purified toxin (poison) causes TSS in a rabbit model that I mentioned was developed in my laboratory. I showed this disease occurred because of massive immune system stimulation and complete dysfunction. That was it then! I discovered the correct toxin. I spent the next four years convincing researchers I was correct— yes, four years—until in 1984 when the toxin was renamed to TSS Toxin, and as the cause of 100 percent of menstrual, vaginal TSS. Woo hoo! I actually knew what I was talking about, and not just blowing smoke. What was I thinking? Do you know how many sleepless nights I had until the code was broken?

I would like to stop a minute and provide an important aside that goes along with risk-taking. Imagine a first-year assistant professor, publicizing a disease that researchers and the biomedical community said did not exist. Imagine also that this same investigator challenged the federal CDC that both vaginal *Staphylococcus aureus* and this toxin PE C were causing the disease. Imagine also that this was in part done on behalf of the American public in the news media. Imagine the harassment by Bruce Dan when I was trying to identify the strains from menstrual, vaginal TSS patients. Then, think about all the sleepless nights I endured, knowing I was correct but still having doubts because few researchers and physicians believed me. That is a lot of weight I was pushing against. It's a good thing I had my wife with whom to talk in order to keep my spirits up during the bleak times. It's also a good thing I had an undergraduate Russell Nishimura to work with in the laboratory. As you will see, he was very important in what we were doing. Just hang on, and you will see.

As I said above, Kathryn Shands was stunned that I was able to identify the TSS *Staphylococcus aureus* and the causative toxin. Several things happened next. First, I told her that there was one *Staphylococcus aureus* strain that produced much more toxin than other isolates. Unfortunately, and with incredibly bad luck, the CDC TSS task force had injected, into the bloodstream of chimpanzees, sterile spent growth medium from this high toxin producer, separated from the *Staphylococcus aureus*. Spent culture medium means that the bacteria had grown as much as they could in this medium, and they had produced their toxins; the CDC separated the culture fluid from the bacteria. They had borrowed the chimpanzees from the Navy. It turned out the one strain that I had said was particularly dangerous because of high amounts of PE C was one that they had injected into a chimpanzee. It killed the chimpanzee. There went $100,000 and a non-human primate.

The next thing that happened was that Dr. Dan arrived at my laboratory, clearly itching for a fight. Kathryn to her great credit brought him up short by saying: "Bruce, he got them all correct. He did it." That was the end of our fighting and the end of my disagreements with the CDC on the cause of menstrual, vaginal TSS. We published on the identification of this toxin in the April 1981 edition of the *Journal of Infectious Diseases*.[8] This became the twelfth most recognized manuscript of all biomedical papers published in journals in the 1980s. The authors in order were Schlievert, Shands, Dan, Schmid, and Nishimura.

The last author on this paper was the undergraduate in my laboratory who helped me test the strains for PE C. Russell Nishimura went on to have a sterling career as a dental school researcher, dentist, and now retiree. He was highly recognized for this contribution by the *Journal of the American Dental Association* and given a scholarship to dental school at UCLA. I thank Russell for his belief in me and what we were doing. In addition to the CDC TSS task force, many folks at UCLA did not believe in menstrual TSS, much less that I could identify a toxin that was causing the disease. Three members of the TSS task force from the CDC were co-authors on the paper describing this brand-new toxin. This is indeed the cause of 100 percent of menstrual TSS, and we know the toxin today as TSS Toxin. By doing statistical analyses, the chance of me finding the correct isolates by chance from the blinded study was:

one chance in one thousand billion, billion, billion, billion, billion. That is a very small likelihood that this was by chance. Thus, my finding the toxin was not an accident; this was indeed the causative toxin.

It was now lunchtime in Los Angeles, and Kathryn asked if we could go have sushi, which we did in the nearby village of Westwood. This was memorable for only one reason. Remember, I was eating with Kathryn Shands and Bruce Dan, two EIS officers from the CDC. Just after we had finished the sushi, Kathryn and I noticed a cockroach crawling across the sushi on the other side of the counter. I chuckle each time I think about it. It could not have been more opportune. We were both disgusted and laughed about it, but fortunately we did not get sick. Kathryn and Bruce then flew back to the CDC in Atlanta.

Soon after this, I realized I could never afford to live in Los Angeles without commuting for one and a half hours each way each day. I also could not afford to buy a home and could not afford to send my planned children to private schools, noting the Los Angeles public school system was a mess at that time. I thus moved to Minnesota and became a faculty member at the University of Minnesota, even taking over the laboratory in which I had trained as a postdoctoral associate. I remained at Minnesota for thirty-one years. I have great friends there! I still hate the cold with a passion. I am well known for complaining that April is supposed to be spring, not the dead of winter. I did get pretty good at broomball—hockey without skates and a ball instead of a puck. I would rather have a surf board and nice warm water.

I need to tell one additional story of what happened early in 1981, late February-early March, prior to publication of my paper in the April edition of the *Journal of Infectious Diseases*. You are likely to say: "No way is this true", but I swear on a stack of bibles it is true as I am telling it. There was another TSS researcher Dr. Merlin Bergdoll, University of Wisconsin, Food Research

Institute, Madison, Wisconsin. Merlin saw himself as a competitor of mine in identifying the toxin associated with this by now much publicized menstrual, vaginal TSS disease. To his credit, Merlin had already identified many of the toxins we call staphylococcal enterotoxins, the causes of millions of cases of food poisoning each year. When you have staphylococcal food poisoning, you are the equivalent of being drunk sick, where you throw up every fifteen minutes for about two days. You think you are going to die, but then you get well with no long-term effects. Merlin worked in the Food Research Institute since staphylococcal enterotoxins do in fact cause lots of food poisoning. He had spent a lifetime (he was already nearing retirement age) trying to get researchers to recognize the great importance of the staphylococcal enterotoxins with some, though minimal success.

Merlin and I became great friends five years later. Late in life Merlin developed aplastic anemia where his bone marrow could no longer produce red blood cells, why is not exactly known. However, one day he called me and said: "Pat, I want you to have all of my staphylococcal strains. I know you will value them and use them to pursue the importance of enterotoxins in human diseases." I gladly accepted receiving the strains, which he immediately sent to me by Federal Express, and which I have even today. I asked Merlin why he did not want to send the strains to his former students. Simply, he said: "I do not trust them scientifically." The night he sent me the strains, Merlin died. The next day one of his daughters called me to tell me that I was the last person to have spoken to Merlin.

She asked, "What did he say?"

I noted that: "Merlin wanted me to have his bacterial strains, with the explanation of why he did not want to send them to others. He said, 'I have not had a lot of contact with my children, but I do love them. I do not think I will live much longer because I am having blood transfusions weekly, and I am not sure how long this can continue. I love my family.'"

Goodbye, Merlin! If you can see us now, you will know that the staphylococcal enterotoxins, notably B and C cause one-half of non-menstrual TSS; we all know this is true. TSS Toxin is the cause of 100 percent of menstrual, vaginal TSS. This family of toxins is the major if not only reason persons die from *Staphylococcus aureus* and Group A streptococci. Staphylococcal enterotoxins A through E types are agents of bioterrorism as decided by the CDC; they were the United States number one bioweapons when we were stock-piling them.

However, I want to go back to the original story I was telling you. One day, out of the blue, Merlin called me; this was when we were competitors and not good friends. He said: "Pat, I understand you have a toxin that you think causes menstrual TSS."

I said: "Yes, I do, and I have a paper in press, ready to be published on the disease."

Merlin asked me the properties of the toxin. He said: "What is the molecular weight of your toxin?"

I knew he was fishing for an answer he did not know, but I did not want to jeopardize my publication with the CDC researchers. I thus told Merlin: "The molecular weight of my toxin is 20,000", knowing it was actually 22,000, close but not exactly right.

Merlin then asked me: "What is the isoelectric point of your toxin?" Again, I was a little bit vague, saying 6.8 when I knew it was 7.2. Again, close but not exact. By the way, isoelectric point is the place from acidic to basic where PE C would have no charge, 7.2 being close to neutrality.

Finally, Merlin asked me: "Can normal skin bacteria like *Staphylococcus epidermidis* make your toxin?" I said yes, but even as of today, not one *Staphylococcus epidermidis* strain has ever been isolated that makes PE C (also known as TSS Toxin). During this phone call, I realized that Merlin was fishing for data so he could try to publish a paper in the scientific literature, ahead of my paper for which I had so many sleepless nights. That is also why I gave him vague information. Merlin did in fact try to have a paper published, ahead of mine in *The Lancet*. What was he thinking? At that time, *The Lancet* was not peer-reviewed, in contrast to the *Journal of infectious Diseases* where my paper had already gone past peer-review, acceptance, and in press for publication. My manuscript was published in April of 1981.

It turns out that *The Lancet* did accept Merlin's manuscript for publication. The paper came out in May 1981,[28] which called his toxin staphylococcal enterotoxin F (SEF). He called it enterotoxin because it shared the property of other staphylococcal enterotoxins of causing vomiting (emesis) when given orally to monkeys and thus, presumably humans. As I will be discussing later, Merlin's toxin was not pure. It was primarily the same as my toxin, but his toxin was contaminated with enterotoxin A, a toxin produced by 80 percent of menstrual TSS isolates of *Staphylococcus aureus*, and this toxin was causing the vomiting Merlin observed in the challenged monkeys. I do not think it is a coincidence that Merlin's publication lists the molecular weight of his toxin as 20,000, the same number I gave him for mine, and a number he never used again. Likewise, he listed this isoelectric point of his toxin as 6.8, the number I gave him, and a number he never used again. Finally, he said *Staphylococcus epidermidis* bacteria could make the toxin. This became a highly controversial topic later with the CDC as will be discussed in detail. However, as I said above, this is mistaken information I gave Merlin in our phone call, and as I said there has never been a *Staphylococcus epidermidis* isolate that produces TSS Toxin.

The publication of these two conflicting stories: PE C versus SEF led to unimaginable symposium debates, often with more than three thousand scientists in the audience at each event. Many scientists tried to "bait" us into squabbling. For example, a researcher from Tufts (now deceased) asked Merlin and me what the properties of our respective toxins were. The Tufts researcher very quickly became sarcastic knowing that the "Midwest dummies" were not as smart as he was. Incidentally, he died at a young age from a massive heart attack. I continued to state the same values as before: molecular weight 22,000, isoelectric point 7.2, and production of toxin restricted to *Staphylococcus aureus* strains able to cause menstrual, vaginal TSS. Then, I noted the toxin is incredibly stable, even when dried onto a Petri dish for a year. However, the toxin in solution turns pale yellow upon storage as a liquid in the refrigerator. Merlin then stated the revised properties of his toxin: 27,000 molecular weight (much higher than before), isoelectric point 8.0 (higher than before), and could be produced by *Staphylococcus epidermidis* (just as he had said before). He said his toxin did not become yellow upon storage. This questioner from Tufts then in a "smart ass" way (high-pitched, little-kid-like) asked: "Well, I wonder where the yellow went", referring to the non-yellow color of Merlin's toxin. I think this was a take-off from a Pepsodent® tooth paste commercial: "You'll wonder where the yellow went, when you brush your teeth with Pepsodent®". I say again, he was being a purposeful "smart ass". This was a National Academy of Sciences, National Academy of Medicine meeting to assess the current knowledge on menstrual TSS. This researcher was instructed to give both Merlin and me a bad time.

By the way, for scientists: The yellow color of my toxin arose over time from the natural formation of yellow Schiff bases between the toxin and the solvent we used to keep the toxin dissolved in water. I also remember when we all were leaving this meeting, one of my postdoctoral mentors (Dr. Louis Wannamaker) saying to me: "Why should a group of National Academy of Medicine researchers, none of whom were studying TSS, have any right to say anything about this disease?" Indeed, I agreed with him, and in fact I wrote a letter to the editor of the *Minneapolis Newspaper* criticizing the conduct of this meeting. The newspaper had written an article addressing the meeting, and I was responding.

It was after a few such squabbles at meetings when I pulled Merlin Bergdoll aside and said: "Merlin, all of these researchers are having a lot of fun watching us fight over the same toxin." Merlin so much wanted these two toxins to be different. But, how could they have been different? I finally convinced Merlin to work with me, and we showed they were in fact the same toxin, and then the research community could not attend symposia to watch Merlin and me battle. Except for one more battle: "What do we call the toxin?" This is addressed in another chapter.

Chapter 7

What are Exotoxins?

I need to spend a chapter speaking about what toxins (poisons) are and how they cause toxic shock syndrome. There are two major kinds of toxins produced by bacteria that cause human diseases. Exotoxins are poisons secreted outside of bacteria and into the tissues of humans, and which are extremely toxic to people; an amount the size of a tenth of a single grain of salt can kill a person. The other kind of toxin is called endotoxin. I mentioned in a prior chapter that microbiologists can tell Gram-positive versus Gram-negative bacteria based on a technique called the Gram-stain where Gram-positive bacteria stain purple, and Gram-negative bacteria stain pink. Both Gram-positive and Gram-negative bacteria can secrete exotoxins into humans, but Gram-positive bacteria are a bit more likely to do this. However, only Gram-negative bacteria have endotoxin.

I will first discuss endotoxin. One kind of bacteria nearly all of us know about is *Escherichia coli*, also known simply as *E. coli*. This kind of bacteria normally lives with us as 1 million per gram of poop; there are 454 grams per pound, so this means 454 million *E. coli* per pound of poop. We have 10 trillion bacteria per gram of poop as a rule. That is a lot of bacteria. However, the majority of them cause us no harm. In contrast, *E. coli* is like *Staphylococcus aureus*, the junk-yard dog that can be mean and nasty under the incorrect circumstances. For example, *E. coli* causes 80 percent of urinary tract infections, commonly seen in women. Additionally, nearly one hundred thousand persons in the United States die each year due to *E. coli*-induced shock. So how do *E. coli* and related bacteria like *Salmonella* and *Shigella* kill people? They use their endotoxin.

Endotoxin is also called lipopolysaccharide, which tells you what it is made of… namely lipids and sugars connected together to form a toxin. Endotoxin is part of the cell of all Gram-negative bacteria and is typically lethal to humans at about one to ten micrograms per human in the bloodstream. Remember that a microgram is about the size of a grain of salt. Yes, humans have injected themselves with one microgram of endotoxin, and they have been admitted to intensive care units in hospitals for two weeks to keep them alive. When you consider swimming in lakes in the summer, the State Health Departments will monitor the coliform count in the lakes. If they find too many *E. coli*, they will advise people not to swim. This is because *E. coli* is a very common cause of disease as noted above.

I mentioned *E. coli* causes a lot of deaths. How does this happen? Endotoxin from the bacteria interacts with immune cells that I have mentioned before, primarily macrophages to cause the production and massive release of small proteins from those macrophages. Those small proteins are called cytokines. The normal role of cytokines is to regulate the body to keep immune function "normal". However, massive production and release of two cytokines have highly negative effects on humans. *E. coli* uses its endotoxin to cause production and release of massive amounts of cytokines called interleukin 1-beta and tumor necrosis factor-alpha. These two molecules together account for *E. coli*-induced shock, or as we many times call it Gram-negative or endotoxin shock. Interleukin 1-beta causes very high fever by direct effects on the hypothalamus part of the brain. This cytokine used to be known as endogenous pyrogen, in that it is produced by our own macrophages, and it causes high fever. The one microgram amount will cause a fever in a human up to 105°F, which is a really high fever.

Tumor necrosis factor-alpha, in high concentrations, causes blood vessels to leak high amounts of fluid into adjacent tissues. The macrophages are not producing tumor necrosis factor-alpha to kill humans. Instead, they would normally cause only modest blood vessel leaking to get blood antibodies into an area of infection. This in turn would help get rid of the bacteria causing the infection.

However, in the immune system, too much of a good thing is usually a really bad thing. Tumor necrosis factor-alpha, causing massive fluid leak into adjacent tissues, leads downstream to failure of proper blood flow, which we call hypotension, and meaning significant drop in blood pressure. Hypotension means not enough oxygen is being transported because blood is not flowing enough. If this gets to be too much of a problem, the organs in the body begin to shut down, and we know this as shock, or in the case of *E. coli*, endotoxin, or Gram-negative shock.

This may seem complicated to you, but all you really need to remember is that interleukin 1-beta causes fever and tumor necrosis factor-alpha causes drop in blood pressure known as hypotension and shock. Later in this chapter, I will explain how fever and hypotension happen in TSS. You will see the similarities. I will also tell you that only some animals, including humans and rabbits as a model for study of the disease, develop TSS.[12] Mice and rats do not. You may ask why this is. Humans and rabbits have lots of these Gram-negative *E. coli*-like bacteria in the intestines, whereas mice and rats do not. Only those animals with lots of *E. coli*-like bacteria develop TSS. Why is this? We simply do not really know. However, I do not think it is a coincidence that endotoxin and TSS Toxin synergize with each other, requiring one million times less of either toxin to kill than when the toxins are present alone.[29]

I am reminded of a patient for whom I was called to help. The patient had a soft tissue abscess that was infected with both *Staphylococcus aureus* and *E. coli*. The *Staphylococcus aureus* was a strain that produced TSS Toxin, but this was not known until later when I tested it. The *E. coli*, as with all *E. coli*, produced endotoxin. Note that we have the situation I mentioned above, the presence of TSS Toxin and endotoxin, so one million increased chance to develop high fever and shock. It also turns out by treating the *E. coli* part of this infection with antibiotics, which is the usual therapy, the killing of *E. coli* results in massive release into the body of endotoxin. This is in the presence of TSS Toxin. What happens is the patient develops shock that cannot be reversed, and the patient dies in a matter of an hour or two. This is exactly what happened to this patient and as well many other patients on whom I acted as a consultant. I offer advice, but the physicians must decide whether or not to take my advice in their treatment options. In the majority of instances, in these dual infections with *E. coli* and *Staphylococcus aureus*, the physicians do not follow my advice, and the patients die. So how would I treat such patients? The first thing I would do is give intravenous immunoglobulin, which always has antibodies against TSS Toxin. These antibodies will neutralize the toxicity of TSS Toxin, and this will prevent the million-fold synergy between TSS Toxin and endotoxin. Then, the abscess can be drained, and antibiotics can be used to treat the infection.

What about Gram-positive bacteria? *Staphylococcus aureus* and *Streptococcus pyogenes* (Group A streptococci) are Gram-positive bacteria that produce exotoxins (secreted poisons), but they do not contain endotoxin. Bacteria like *Escherichia coli* (*E. coli*) and *Salmonella* contain endotoxin as a part of them.

For this book, we are primarily concerned with exotoxin poisons. They are the most potent toxins (poisons) known. I mentioned *Staphylococcus aureus* and Group A streptococci produce exotoxins. But, so do *Clostridium tetani*, *Clostridium botulinum*, and *Corynebacterium diphtheriae*. The names of these latter three bacteria tell you what they cause. *Clostridium tetani* causes tetanus or lock jaw. The muscles controlling the jaw are used a lot and are very strong. People with tetanus have their jaws locked in the contracted form and cannot un-contract. This causes them to have a sneering type grin (called sardonic), and at the same time, they throw their heads back. They further constrict neck and back muscles, which cannot be un-constricted. This causes the patients to break their backs and die. This is why we vaccinate against tetanus every eight to ten years… to be sure you have strong immunity, in the form of protective antibodies, in case you step on a rusty nail or have other trauma that implants the bacteria into you. *Clostridium botulinum* causes botulism, associated with eating certain canned foods. The exotoxin produced by *Clostridium botulinum* has the opposite effect of tetanus toxin in that the muscles lose the ability to contract. Your ability to breathe depends on muscle contraction, and failure to allow you to breathe results in death. The effects of botulism toxin can remain in place for months. This is the reason you do not eat canned foods that have bulges in the cans. And yes, this is the same toxin that is injected into people to help un-wrinkle the person's skin. The amounts injected into people are extremely small. We do not vaccinate against botulism as a disease since the botulism is very rare.

Corynebacterium diphtheriae are Gram-positive bacteria that make diphtheria toxin (poison). This toxin kills cells in the throats of victims and kills heart cells to stop the hearts from beating. Just like for scarlet fever, there used to be separate wings of hospitals to isolate persons with diphtheria. It was a major killer in its time. Now, we vaccinate against diphtheria. This is the "D" part of the DaPT vaccine (diphtheria-whooping cough-tetanus) that we all receive six times before starting kindergarten. We vaccinate with biologically non-toxic variants of the toxins to stimulate protective antibodies.

Each of the above toxins (tetanus, botulism, and diphtheria) are enzymes that destroy important components of our cells, ultimately causing the death of the person.

For the complete purists among you, the exact mechanism of action of diphtheria toxin, for example, is to inhibit protein synthesis in our cells. Proteins are made from the enormous number of genes in each of our cells. Thus, protein synthesis is a critical activity in our cells. The machinery in our cells to encode proteins from genes is complex, with all kinds of protein factors required. One of these factors is called elongation factor 2, and this factor itself has an unusual amino acid called diphthamide. I wonder why? We also have a lot of a molecules in our cells required for normal metabolism. One of these molecules is called nicotinamide adenine dinucleotide, or as we call it NAD. The action of diphtheria toxin is to cleave NAD into nicotinamide and ADP-ribose. The toxin then binds irreversibly the ADP-ribose to the diphthamide amino acid in elongation factor 2. The effect of this enzymatic function is to inhibit protein synthesis in the cell. One molecule of diphtheria toxin can inhibit 90 percent of all protein synthesis in our cells; this kills our cells. The other two toxins I mentioned above, tetanus and botulism toxins, are both proteases cleaving into small pieces proteins that are important components of nerve transmission. Not only these three toxins, but most toxins are enzymes, for example cholera toxin, the toxin that causes traveler's diarrhea, the toxin that causes hemolytic uremic syndrome, pertussis (whooping cough) toxin, and the two toxins that cause anthrax.

As noted in the prior chapter, I discovered staphylococcal PE C, later known as TSS Toxin, in 1980, and I published the definitive study on this toxin in April 1981.[8] So... how does this toxin work? It has absolutely no enzyme function. Weird, huh? The toxin works by binding and over-activating two kinds of cells of our immune system. Because the toxin has no enzyme function, the poison must be present in higher concentrations in the body than enzymes. Enzymes cleave things and then can cleave things again and again. TSS Toxin binds to cells, and to bind to all target cells, it simply takes more toxin than an enzyme.

As a brief summary from a prior chapter, there are four major kinds of immune cells. The ones that we first see at infection sites and that make up the major kinds of white blood cells are called neutrophils or polymorphonuclear leukocytes (PMNs). They make up 70 percent of our white blood cells, and they are the markers of inflammation. TSS Toxin has no direct effect on these cells. However, PMN migrate to infection sites, as they are supposed to do, and their functions are blocked by the production and action of cytokines by other immune cells. Thus, relatively few of these PMN cells come into the area of *Staphylococcus aureus* infection due to TSS Toxin. This biological activity not only prevents these PMN cells from doing their jobs, but this also reduces the ability of physicians to see signs of infection, because of relative lack of inflammation as mentioned in prior chapters.

The next three kinds of immune cells make up 30 percent of your immune system, with each cell type being 10 percent of the white blood cells. The first of these is called B lymphocytes. These cells are responsible for making antibodies that give you immunity to toxins and some bacteria. If you make a graph of the amount of antibodies against TSS Toxin versus age, there is a straight line from no antibodies at three months of age to a significant amount of antibodies in 80 percent of people by age twelve; this was shown conclusively by two acquaintances of mine, Drs. Jim Vergeront from Madison Wisconsin,[10] and Jeffrey Parsonnet from Dartmouth-Hitchcock Medical Center in New Hampshire,[30] and their colleagues. The amounts of antibodies formed and present in the bloodstream of these 80 percent of persons prevents TSS due to TSS Toxin by binding to the toxin and neutralizing its toxic activity. The remaining 20 percent of folks who do not develop antibodies by age twelve will never develop antibodies. These are the people, including menstruating women, who may develop TSS due to TSS Toxin. Even as of today as I write, it is not clear what disease children develop until all 80 percent have protective antibodies by twelve years of age.

I think it is also important to keep in mind that there are fifty million women of menstrual age in the United States. Even though 80 percent will develop antibodies to protect them from TSS Toxin, 20 percent will not ever develop antibodies and thus, will never have antibodies. This is ten million women… which is a lot of susceptible folks. It is also not clear why those 20 percent of women do not develop antibodies. We are all exposed at some time to TSS Toxin-producing *Staphylococcus aureus*, yet 20 percent of us do not develop antibodies. Jeff Parsonnet and I have developed quick, easy tests to measure whether or not twelve-year-olds do or do not have antibodies to TSS Toxin. Our thinking was that if all twelve-year-olds are tested, we can identify the 20 percent who do not develop antibodies. Those young women can be advised never to use tampons. We thought this test could be run upon the first appearance of menstrual periods and first visits to their gynecologists. This test never got off the ground because companies said: "The incidence of menstrual TSS is not high enough to make this a commercial enterprise." They completely missed the point. What were they thinking? When young women develop menstrual TSS, we then already know they do not and never will have antibodies to TSS Toxin. The importance of the test we wanted used is that there are enormous numbers of women who could have this test to tell if they are at risk. At this time, the development of the test for commercial use is not being done. I occasionally run the test on my laboratory folks and friends who ask, but routinely I do not do the test.

There are two kinds of immune cells that remain, each at 10 percent of our white blood cells. Both of these cell types are the principal targets of TSS Toxin: T lymphocytes and macrophages. T lymphocytes are the brilliant cells of the immune system in that they are designed to tell all other adaptive immune cells what to do. Normally, when we encounter something foreign, one in ten thousand of our T lymphocytes will become activated and either tell B cells to make antibodies, get rid of some bacteria, viruses, and fungi by themselves, or tell macrophages to kill bacteria. They do this by again making small protein molecules called cytokines that act on other immune cells, mostly to activate them. From this interaction, there is a well-controlled immune response, and we develop immunity in about four days.

However, TSS Toxin bypasses this normal response to cause an abnormal interaction. This leads to activation of 10 percent of all of our T lymphocytes.[31] These activated T lymphocytes divide and become up to 70 percent of all T lymphocytes in TSS patients. This is way, way, way too many T lymphocytes. The reason is that they then are programmed to produce way, way, way too many cytokines. One of the most important cytokines produced is called interferon gamma. This cytokine activates macrophages. Because there is now way, way, way too much interferon gamma, way, way, way too many macrophages become activated. This tremendous activation of macrophages results in their production of additional cytokines. Two of these are very important, as I have mentioned before. The first is called interleukin 1-beta or endogenous pyrogen (fever producing agent). Interelukin1-beta is the molecule that causes fever, one of the major defining features of TSS. The second cytokine is tumor necrosis factor-alpha (a.k.a. cachectin, meaning wasting away). Tumor necrosis factor-alpha has its major effect on the blood vessels causing them to leak. Leaky vessels as mentioned above causes a dramatic drop in blood pressure in TSS, also known as hypotension, which may progress to shock when organs shut down and unfortunately to some deaths as well. This dramatic drop in blood pressure is a major defining property of menstrual, vaginal TSS.

The next set of symptoms of TSS are the sunburn-like rash and skin peeling if the patient survives. As I mentioned before, this rash is also scarlet fever-like. Most women who develop menstrual toxic shock syndrome will tell you that they had at least one prior episode of TSS without a rash, prior to having the full-blown disease with rash. In our studies, the rash occurs as a result of allergy to TSS Toxin.

Let me remind you of poison ivy, where the rash is the result of the same kind of allergy. The first time you are exposed to poison ivy you do not get that itchy, vesicular (sterile blisters) rash. The second or third time is when the rash and vesicles occur. The same is true with TSS and by the same mechanism. The rash is actually the result of too much interferon gamma.

I am now reminded of the Arlo Guthrie song "Alice's Restaurant", where a litterbug wants to go into the military to go to Vietnam, during the war, and "kill, kill, kill". This is what interferon-activated macrophages want to do: "kill, kill, kill". In doing so, they damage the patient's skin and mucous membranes, causing her to turn red, like sunburn-damage to skin. You may listen to Arlo Guthrie's song at https://www.youtube.com/watch?v=m57gzA2JCcM. When patients succumb to menstrual TSS, autopsies have been performed to find sites of damage. The skin and mucous membranes are clearly damaged by the allergic response of macrophages, but also those same activated macrophages kill the patient's own red blood cells and platelets. I mentioned platelet destruction before when I asked the CDC if this dramatic fall in platelet numbers would stay low, as in autoimmune thrombocytopenic purpura. When the macrophages stop being so highly activated by interferon gamma, as in when the patient recovers from her disease, the platelet numbers return to normal.

So where does the skin peeling come from? The allergic reaction can lead to skin peeling just like you see in poison ivy. However, in TSS, large areas of skin can peel, much more than would be expected simply due to poison ivy. I think this happens when the patient recovers and the swelling (edema) goes away, leaving a lot of loose skin... which is skin that peels. Remember, tumor necrosis factor-alpha causes blood vessel leak, with fluid escaping into the tissues. Our largest tissue is skin and mucous membranes, with lots of blood vessels to leak. Indeed, menstrual TSS patients can swell up like the Michelin® tire man (woman). This happens because physicians treat patients with up to fifteen liters (quarts) per day of fluid to keep blood pressure in the normal range—that is, to keep the patient alive. So, when the patient recovers, she still has a lot of fluid to eliminate, which she does by peeing. The blood vessels close up with no more fluid leaking into tissues. The patient now has a lot of loose skin to peel.

There is one other component of menstrual TSS called the variable multi-organ component. This means that many organs can be affected but variably so. One of these mentioned above is a very significant drop in platelets. Platelets allow you to clot to prevent chronic bleeding problems. The platelets are being eaten massively by the macrophages that have become too activated by T lymphocytes.[18] Macrophages are not particularly smart, so they attack as their major function. In a normal immune response to infection, these cells are under control but not in menstrual toxic shock syndrome.

Vomiting and diarrhea are the most common early symptoms of TSS, and with fever, has led to the disease being described as and confused with "the flu". Nearly all TSS *Staphylococcus aureus* bacteria produce other toxins called enterotoxins, as I mentioned in another chapter. For example, 80 percent of menstrual TSS strains produce enterotoxin A, the most common cause of

Dr. Patrick M. Schlievert

staphylococcal food poisoning, defined by vomiting and diarrhea commencing two to eight hours after exposure to the enterotoxin. These agents act on a patient's vagus nerve, the flight-or-fight nerve. This nerve controls lots of things in the body, including symptoms of panic attacks, the incredible strength of some folks during high stress, and nausea and vomiting responses of the intestinal tract. Many patients with TSS come to the hospital Emergency Department or their Urgent Care Center with a few days of vomiting and diarrhea. If particularly dehydrated, they are given a liter (quart) of fluid and sent home. Some are simply told to go home, that they have the flu. All are told if symptoms persist to phone back in and schedule an appointment. Many of these patients go home, go to bed because they do not feel well, and do not wake up. They die in bed because of the shock of menstrual TSS. The peak onset of menstrual TSS is day four of menstruation. This means the patient develops increasing flu-like symptoms through day three, and then all hell breaks loose on day four, or while the patient is sleeping... she simply never wakes.

I have participated in unexplained death projects. It is my estimate that as many as 30 percent of unexplained deaths are due to the various forms of TSS. It is only in the last few years that in the world I alone have been able to measure TSS Toxin in human patients. Since 1980, I have been able to measure the lack of antibodies in TSS patients. Putting these two together, I am now able to tell if someone died of TSS.

Let me tell you about a recent patient who died while being transported by helicopter to the regional hospital. In the autopsy, TSS Toxin-producing *Staphylococcus aureus* was isolated from multiple body sites. I made that determination. I also showed the patient had eight hundred micrograms (eight thousand lethal doses) of TSS Toxin in her body, and she lacked antibodies to TSS Toxin. What do you think killed her? Interleukin 1-beta and tumor necrosis factor-alpha!

I will tell you another tragic story. A woman went to her local Medical Clinic because she had vomiting and diarrhea. What do nurses do as the first thing when you are seen in a clinic? They take your pulse, blood pressure, and temperature. The Clinic forgot to do this. How is that even possible? What were they thinking? The nurses also noted that the patient staggered when she walked. I should note that the reduction in blood pressure that we know as hypotension can be seen as dizziness upon standing, called orthostatic hypotension. This would make the patient stagger. That night, the patient died of TSS. I made that determination from the presence of TSS Toxin *Staphylococcus aureus*, the lack of protective antibodies, and the presence of TSS Toxin in the patient: one thousand micrograms (ten thousand lethal doses). It is nice that I can do these things, don't you think? It would be even nicer if they were done prior to the patient dying, so perhaps the patient can be saved.

There are major liver, kidney, muscle, and brain toxic effects. For many of these, such as the brain effects I mentioned in a prior chapter, even today we do not know why they occur. I will mention quickly one other multi-organ change that we see all the time but is poorly understood: extreme muscle soreness and tetany (extreme muscle contraction). This effect is seen by the rise in the blood of a human enzyme called creatinine phosphokinase (CPK). This rise in concentration in the blood may be very great. There may be so much muscle damage and tetany that women with menstrual TSS will not be able to get out of bed. They are extremely sore. In fact, they may urinate and poop right in bed instead of making it to the bathroom.

Another way to think about CPK is to think of marathon runners. Upon completion of their first marathons, the next day, runners will go down stairs backwards, because their leg muscles become so sore from lactic acid build-up and muscle damage. The muscle damage causes astronomical elevations of CPK. Indeed, some of the first marathoners were thought to be having heart attacks, since CPK levels rise dramatically also due to heart muscle damage. It turns out that the major source of the elevated CPK in marathon runners is the leg and butt muscles. Those of us who run marathons know that the order of gaining energy during running is first glycogen (sugar) stores, then muscle, and finally fat; wouldn't it be nice to lose the fat before the muscle? It is likely that at some prehistoric time, it was necessary to conserve fat as much as possible for lean times that may arise, and this may have selected the order of energy gain.

Along with the highly elevated CPK, we see a very dramatic drop in blood levels of the metal, calcium. When calcium levels drop too low, we see the symptoms of tetanus or dramatic, unrelenting contraction of muscles. This may in fact contribute to the elevated CPK. However, we do not know why calcium levels drop so dramatically. After all these years, it seems like we should know, but we do not.

I want to tell you one other funny-sad story here. About five years ago a physician from Texas called me. He was really excited because he thought he had found a new toxin that caused menstrual TSS. He had two young women with menstrual TSS, where he had of course isolated two *Staphylococcus aureus* strains. He had sent the two strains to a reference laboratory in California to test them for production of TSS Toxin. This laboratory was CLIA (Clinical Laboratory Improvement Amendments) -certified, which is a requirement for performance of diagnostic tests. My laboratory is not CLIA-certified because my major activities are research and teaching, not diagnostic testing. Thus, any diagnostic testing I do is strictly for research purposes. So, this CLIA-certified laboratory performed the test and found the two *Staphylococcus aureus* strains to be TSS Toxin-negative. This is what led the physician to call me. He had two strains from young women with menstrual TSS where TSS Toxin was not being produced. We had a conversation to be sure the patients indeed had menstrual TSS, and then he sent me the two strains. Being appropriately cynical, I decided the first thing I should do is test the two strains for ability to produce TSS Toxin; I have seen too many mistakes in my time as a researcher. As I expected, both strains produced TSS Toxin; there was no new toxin. Even today, there is only one toxin that causes menstrual TSS, namely TSS Toxin. I called the physician and told him the result, which of course was disappointing to him. No new toxin discovery. However, we both discussed how the reference laboratory in California, which is CLIA-certified, did not find TSS Toxin, but I did. Thus, he was not quite on board with my test result. So, he called the California laboratory. They told him that he should believe my result, that they did not have faith in their test, and indeed, that they use me as their reference laboratory. Subsequent testing showed that my result was the correct result for the two strains.

Thus, we know now that TSS Toxin binds to T lymphocytes and macrophages, and the binding of these two cells together leads to the symptoms of TSS. However, I mentioned that there is something called streptococcal toxic shock syndrome, and *Streptococcus pyogenes* (Group A streptococci) do not produce TSS Toxin. Additionally, in a prior chapter I also said that staphylococcal enterotoxins B and C cause 50 percent of non-menstrual TSS. How can this be?

I proposed in my first National Institutes of Health grant to study TSS Toxin which reportedly did not exist and that caused a disease that reportedly did not exist. I indicated there are toxins related to TSS Toxin, produced by both *Staphylococcus aureus* and Group A streptococci. I was not believed! Indeed, I was told by the grant review panel that there was no evidence that the staphylococcal and streptococcal toxins were in any way related. They said that if I wanted to study them separately, that was fine, but then I had to apply for two grants instead of one. This was at a time (1980) when I was not allowed to publish a manuscript describing streptococcal TSS; it was not until 1987 that my first collaborative publication came out on streptococcal TSS in the *New England Journal of Medicine*.[13]

My thoughts were: Let's see, we have two families of toxins that have mostly the same biological activities, cause the same kind of disease, have the same ability to cause fever, hypotension, and sunburn-like rash, and can be purified by using the same harsh methods. Scarlet fever toxin A from Group A streptococci and staphylococcal enterotoxins B and C are even similar in reactivity to antibodies. I applied for the study of the toxins as separate families, and after ten additional years finally convinced the grant review panel that the families were in fact one and the same family.

We know today that there is a large family of these related toxins, and today we call them pyrogenic toxin superantigens. I had called them pyrogenic toxins since they are the most potent pyrogens (fever-causing agents) known. In 1990, Drs. Philippa Marrack and John Kappler determined the molecular basis for the cross-bridging of T lymphocytes and macrophages and in their paper called them superantigens.[32] The superantigen name stuck for the large family.

Here is what we know today. TSS Toxin causes 100 percent of menstrual toxic shock syndrome and 50 percent of nonmenstrual staphylococcal TSS, including the 100 percent fatal cases in childhood influenza-associated toxic shock syndrome. Staphylococcal enterotoxin types B and C cause 50 percent of nonmenstrual staphylococcal TSS. The streptococcal scarlet fever toxins types A and C cause nearly all cases of streptococcal TSS. And yes... all of these toxins look very similar when you look at them at the molecular level, but immunity to them is usually fairly specific. Only 80 percent of us ever develop immunity to any given one of these toxins, and this happens by age twelve. Some of us have immunity to one of the pyrogenic toxin superantigens, some of us have immunity to more than one, but all of us lack immunity to at least one of these toxins. These toxins are a major if not the only reason *Staphylococcus aureus* and *Streptococcus pyogenes* kill humans.

For the purists among you, we even know the structure of each of these toxins down at the molecular level, and we even know the exact nature of their interactions with T lymphocytes and macrophages. Much of this work was done by my laboratory in collaboration with Dr. Roy Mariuzza, University of Maryland and Dr. John McCormick, University of Western Ontario.[33,34,35,36,37,38,39,40] I have always thought that Roy Mariuzza merits a Nobel Prize for his impressive contributions here and in immune cell molecular structures. Roy is unusual but exceptionally bright. He started to go to medical school but decided this was not for him, so he went on to obtain a PhD instead. This is backward of what many scientists have done.

Each of these pyrogenic toxin superantigens is about ten thousand times smaller than the bacteria that produce them. In inches they are about twelve millionth by twenty millionth of an inch (width and length) looking like very small kidneys. They are composed entirely of amino acids, which are connected together into proteins that are very tightly folded outside bacterial cells into the kidney bean shape. It is that very tight folding that makes them very resistant to degradation by acids and heat. For example, staphylococcal enterotoxins are not degraded by our stomach acid, giving them time to pass through the stomach and stimulate the vagus nerve to cause vomiting and diarrhea. Likewise, the toxins are quite resistant to degradation by bleach. I will talk about this property more in a later chapter.

We even know the precise structures of the pyrogenic toxin superantigens with their interaction partner on T lymphocytes, the T lymphocyte receptor, and on macrophages, the molecules that help determine how we initiate adaptive immune responses in the first place. I will say that if I was a bacterium and wanted to cause problems in humans, I would want to mess up the immune system in the same way these toxins do.

I now want to tell you an odd but interesting and "telling" story about studies of these pyrogenic toxin superantigens.

I think we will all know that throughout history, microorganisms, usually bacteria, have changed the course of history. For example, the Religious Crusaders and Napoleon's Army were decimated by epidemic typhus, caused by the bacteria *Rickettsia prowazekii*. In some storming of castles and walled cities, it was sometimes a good idea to catapult diseased dead bodies, for example those who died of pneumonic plague, over the castle or city walls to try to kill the residents through terrible infections. In the 1300s and again in the 1600s, nearly 40 percent of Europe was killed by bubonic and pneumonic plagues. As we come closer to home, we remember the anthrax scare after September 11, 2001 in the United States when anthrax spores were shipped through the mail and resulted in deadly anthrax in several individuals.

My postdoctoral mentor at the University of Minnesota, Dr. Dennis Watson, performed research for the United States Federal Government during World War II. His job was to develop vaccines against typhus and anthrax. He accomplished both of these objectives by working for Naval Medical Research Unit (NAMRU) 4. This was research designed to protect our soldiers against deadly diseases that had been threatened for use by the Axis Powers in the form of biological weapons.

An important question arises: Did the United States develop its own offensive, as opposed to defensive, weapons? The answer is definitely yes! What is likely to surprise you is what those weapons were. The number one biowarfare (biological) weapon of the United States was the pyrogenic toxin superantigen, staphylococcal enterotoxin B, that causes highly fatal, non-menstrual TSS when aerosolized into the lungs. It has been documented that each year in the 1950s and 1960s, our country stockpiled five to six tons per year. Keep in mind that we know that an amount as small as one-tenth of a grain of salt is lethal in humans. In comparison, five to six tons is an enormous amount.

So why are pyrogenic toxin superantigens such good bioweapons? The answer is simple. They are easy to produce in massive amounts. They are incredibly toxic. They do not inactivate easily in the environment. They do not require processing (referred to as weaponizing) for use as weapons.

I have been asked what I thought would happen if a pound of staphylococcal enterotoxin B was placed in the food court of the Mall of America in Bloomington, Minnesota. I used to give seminars about this scenario, so this is not some national security secret. It is important to keep in mind that at the time I was asked to speak, there were more visitors to the Mall of America per year than Disney World. I estimated that the first day of exposure, one thousand persons would develop fatal pulmonary (lung) TSS. This number would continue to rise over the next few days until the Minnesota Department of Health stepped in to close the mall. The first day, there would be over fifty thousand people with vomiting and diarrhea lasting forty-eight hours, as this toxin orally causes staphylococcal food poisoning. This would also continue to increase for a few additional days, and there would be fifty thousand people the first day with purulent pink eye caused by the toxin. And to think, we do not even recognize that this latter disease exists, even today. The net effect would be to shut down the Mall of America until it could be cleaned up.

How do you clean it up? Pyrogenic toxin superantigens are all incredibly stable. They can withstand boiling for an hour. The acid and enzymes in your stomach indeed make them more active. Lye is the major thing that will destroy them. That is what would be required to clean up the mess, and it is an enormous mall contaminated with an incredibly toxic toxin.

You think something like this could never happen? That it is out of the question? Consider this. In the 1990s an East Coast newspaper published an article that the mafia in a major city felt it was losing money due to insider theft. Some "bright mafia bulb" got the idea: "Let's get some staphylococcal enterotoxin B and contaminate our money with it. Whoever gets sick are the ones stealing our money." This was in fact done. The problem was, non-mafia folks started developing forty-eight hours of vomiting and diarrhea from the money entering the general circulation at cash registers and banks, with people handling this contaminated money and then touching their mouths.

I have been working with these toxins since 1976, and as noted above I described TSS Toxin in April 1981, which is the most toxic of the pyrogenic toxin superantigens to humans. In two weeks, I can easily make a pound of TSS Toxin. Because of this, I decided in 1985 that these toxins needed to be controlled more carefully in my laboratory and indeed, kept away from potential terrorists. At that time, I was setting up to collaborate on determining the molecular structures of the toxins and in combination with T lymphocyte and macrophage receptors. To do this, I had to prepare very large amounts. What I did then was change all the locks on my laboratory door, making my laboratory so secure that even the University President could not gain access. Only my personnel and the police could enter. We did not even allow custodians to enter. In effect, only folks with the need to have access were allowed to enter. This was fifteen years before the 2001 anthrax scare. When the anthrax scare happened, the CDC finally established new rules for the study of these toxins. My laboratory was being watched like a hawk until about three years ago. Incredibly, at that time, the CDC verbally stated that I was the most serious threat to the health and safety of Americans of anyone at the University of Iowa. When I confronted them about this, they disavowed any knowledge of someone making such a statement. Multiple people at the University of Iowa heard it said though. When I was at the University of Minnesota, periodically members of the FBI would ask other faculty members what they thought of me and my mental stability. I was not then and never have been a threat.

I remember one day there was a problem with our door lock at the University of Minnesota. To show you how I felt, I slept in front of the door, on the inside, blocking all entrance to the laboratory. This was done until the lock could be fixed. I am a danger to the American public? I THINK NOT!

I should also tell you a story about cloning the pyrogenic toxin superantigen genes. I was into genetic cloning on the ground floor, long before there were even university courses to teach students how to clone genes. Today, such cloning is trivial, but it was not in the early years. Back in 1980, I asked the federal Recombinant DNA Advisory Committee, called RAC, for permission to clone streptococcal scarlet fever toxin A, one of the pyrogenic toxin superantigens. After a month of consideration, they gave me permission, so long as I cloned the toxin gene into a heavily mutated strain of *E. coli*, one that could not survive in nature. I was told by the biomedical science community that this cloning would be impossible to accomplish since I was crossing an important bacterial barrier, Gram-positive into Gram-negative. In fact, this was so trivial, even I was amazed. To my knowledge, this was the first toxin of any sort that was cloned.[41] The reason I could do this is that I had a graduate student, now Dr. Lane Johnson, who could do any kind of genetic experiment with the greatest of skill. Lane went on to work in industry, having an incredible career until he retired two years ago. This cloning ultimately led to us cloning many other pyrogenic toxin superantigens, including the gene for TSS Toxin. This then ultimately allowed my laboratory folks to introduce mutations in the genes to make the toxins for vaccinating people but not toxic to people. Indeed, an Austrian group has now done the first human trial of vaccination against TSS Toxin.[42] Why not me? I have not been able to obtain funding from the National Institutes of Health for doing such experiments... as good as they would be for the American public. I am told such experiments are not innovative enough to merit funding. Just three months ago I received notice that my grant application to the National Institutes of Health for cross-vaccination against both *Staphylococcus aureus* and Group A streptococci was not of enough interest even to be in the top one-third of applications. What were they thinking? Certainly, they were not thinking of human health as innovative research.

Chapter 8

August–September 1980;
More Important Than Ever

Now, back to the menstrual, vaginal toxic shock syndrome story. The two most important months in the menstrual TSS epidemic were August and September 1980. August is important because of a meeting called for and held by the CDC in Atlanta, Georgia. Several of us as TSS researchers were invited to attend. I remember the CDC TSS task force members obviously were present, as were Drs. Jim Todd (Denver Children's Hospital) Michael Osterholm (Minnesota State Epidemiologist and Head of the Tri-State TSS Study [Minnesota, Wisconsin, and Iowa], Jeffrey Davis (Wisconsin State Epidemiologist), and me. In addition, the CDC invited two Procter & Gamble scientists, represented by researchers Drs. Roger Stone, whom I mentioned previously, and Owen Carter. No other tampon manufacturers were invited, as the CDC had decided Rely® tampons were the major if not only risk factor for menstrual TSS. It quickly became clear to me that this was a meeting set up to pressure Procter & Gamble to remove Rely® tampons from the market.

The CDC presented their case, finding epidemiologically that the cause of the menstrual TSS epidemic was almost exclusively Rely® tampons. This fit perfectly with biased studies, based largely on Dr. Bruce Dan standing beside and pointing to a display of Rely® tampons in San Francisco, and then advising women with menstrual TSS to notify the CDC. Their presentation also fit perfectly with their epidemiology curve which showed a highly significant rise in menstrual TSS cases with the initiation of Rely® tampon sales. It was clear to me from my time at UCLA, and to other non-CDC epidemiologists that although Rely® tampons were significantly associated with menstrual, so were other high-absorbency tampons.

I remember multiple problems during this meeting. First as mentioned above, CDC epidemiologists performed their initial study in the face of the publicity that originated from my laboratory at UCLA. One member of the CDC toxic shock syndrome task force had come to the San Francisco area, and he stood, pointing to a display of Rely® tampons, asking that if women had menstrual toxic shock syndrome, that they report these cases to the CDC. The fact that he stood pointing to a display of Rely® tampons made it 100 percent certain that the CDC would find an unusually high association with that tampon brand. Women who developed menstrual TSS while using other high-absorbency tampons were not as encouraged to report cases. As I was at the UCLA Medical Center, I spoke often with the Los Angeles County Health Department officials. We knew, based on reports of cases to the Health Department, that all high-absorbency tampons were associated and not just Rely® brand tampons. Our observations fit with the highest quality epidemiology study on menstrual TSS, the Tri-State TSS Study. Their study published in 1982 recognized that risk of toxic shock syndrome correlated with absorbency of tampons, with higher absorbency more associated than low absorbency.[5] It is thus no coincidence that the CDC TSS task force found epidemiologically that menstrual TSS was associated with Rely® tampons, based on their mode of operation.

The second problem with the CDC meeting was that the chief of the CDC TSS task force pulled me aside at a coffee break, and she stated: "Pat, we know the epidemic is caused by the sale of Rely® tampons." I pointed out that menstrual TSS cases were associated with all tampons of high absorbency and not just Rely® tampons. This comment was scoffed at as irrelevant. I also stated that there was another kind of TSS, caused by *Streptococcus pyogenes* (Group A streptococci). This comment was also summarily ignored. You will note that I have previously mentioned streptococcal TSS multiple times, and I will again in detail later. It was not until 1987 in the *New England Journal of Medicine* that Dr. Larry Cone and I published a case description of streptococcal TSS.[13] This was followed by the "gold standard" publication of cases, diagnostic criteria, and treatment by Drs. Dennis Stevens, Edward Kaplan, and me as the lead article in a 1989 *New England Journal of Medicine*.[14]

The third problem was the CDC TSS task force was populated by multiple young epidemiologists, including Drs. Kathryn Shands and Bruce Dan, the Chief and Deputy Chief, respectively. They had only minimal experience in performance of required national epidemiology studies. Additionally, they lacked significant knowledge of the disease-causing abilities of *Staphylococcus aureus* and Group A streptococci.

It is also critical to note that Director of the CDC at that time, Dr. William Foege, had been called to a senate subcommittee meeting in June 1980, chaired by Senator Ted Kennedy. The senator was investigating toxic waste, but he now wanted to know what this menstrual TSS was. Dr. Foege explained the disease and importantly, that he would have the problem solved by the end of 1980. This last point, of having the problem solved by the end of 1980 was a major problem, namely, promising a senator that TSS would be solved by the end of the year. I would never tell a senator, particularly one with such influence, that I would guarantee the solution in less than six months. Science, even for the CDC, does not function that rapidly.

In the face of this knowledge, it is no wonder that the CDC TSS task force told the two Procter & Gamble representatives at the meeting that their tampon, Rely® brand, was THE problem, and they should remove the tampon from the market. CDC could not force removal, but they could use their federal influence to make it happen anyway. Procter & Gamble did indeed remove the Rely® tampons from the market. What were the consequences of this directive and pressure by CDC?

First and simply, women no longer had access to Rely® tampons. Many women stated to me that Rely® tampons were the best tampons that they had ever used. Now we know that 80 percent of young women twelve years of age and older already have antibodies that protect them from menstrual TSS. Rely® tampons would have been perfectly safe for their use; unfortunately, we did not know this at the time. I trust these women with their glowing statements about Rely® tampons, do not know about the army of researchers available to Procter & Gamble to make such a "perfect" tampon available to consumers.

Second, women who used Rely® tampons often changed to use of other high-absorbency tampons, thinking they were now safe since CDC made the association with Rely® tampons. In 1984, there was a menstrual TSS case that was tried in court in Kansas City, Missouri. The judge in that case told International Playtex that if they removed polyacrylate rayon from their tampons, used to make them high absorbency, the judge would reduce the plaintiff punitive award from $10 million to $1.35 million. Playtex and then Tambrands removed the polyacrylate rayon from tampons, making only relatively low absorbency tampons available for use by women. If you make the calculation: the fatality rate for menstrual, vaginal TSS as determined by the CDC was 30 percent at that time. Then, from the time Rely® tampons were removed from the market in August 1980, until all high-absorbency tampons were removed from the market in 1984, an additional six thousand women in the United States likely succumbed (died) due to menstrual TSS. This could have been avoided if the Tri-State TSS Study was valued by the CDC at that time. It is also important to note that Kimberly Clark also marketed high-absorbency tampons, but at the first hint of associated TSS cases, they removed those tampons from the market voluntarily. Kimberly Clark is most known for marketing menstrual pads, and they did not want to jeopardize those sales.

Other important things happened after the removal of Rely® tampons from the market. Until September 1980, the number of cases of menstrual TSS reported to the CDC rose, but after removal of Rely® tampons from the market, the number of cases went down dramatically, leading to an often-cited curve of cases shown by the CDC. The CDC belief was indeed that they had solved the menstrual TSS problem before the end of 1980 as promised by Dr. Foege. The problem with this was that in September 1980, the CDC stopped doing active surveillance to find menstrual TSS cases. It is well known that active surveillance is the only way to know the truest number of cases. Although not perfect, it is immensely better than doing passive surveillance. Active surveillance means that physicians are required to report cases to the Health Departments, who in turn report cases to the CDC.

Passive surveillance means that physicians are left to decide if they will report cases. This type of surveillance will result in fewer than 10 percent of cases reported. Physicians are incredibly busy and thus, report cases most often only when required to do so.

How do we know if I am correct on the effect of changes in the CDC reporting of cases from active to passive surveillance? The "gold standard" epidemiology study was the Tri-State TSS Study, published in 1982, led by the epidemiologists at Minnesota, Wisconsin, and Iowa.[5] They continued to perform active surveillance after removal of Rely® from the market. This study found that cases did NOT change when Rely® tampons were removed from the market. All that happened was that women changed to other high-absorbency tampons, and they continued to develop life-threatening menstrual TSS. It was not until the lawsuit discussed above in 1984 that total menstrual cases were reduced in number.

I know of two other things which the CDC did in this time period. One, when I applied to have my National Institutes of Health grant renewed to study menstrual, vaginal TSS, the CDC TSS task force was present at the grant review panel. It is no surprise to me then that my grant was not renewed. Keep in mind that I had described the *Staphylococcus aureus* toxin, TSS Toxin (then called pyrogenic exotoxin C; PE C) causing menstrual TSS, I had shown why tampons were associated (the introduction of oxygen [air] within tampons), and I had described that most useful animal model to study how the disease occurred. I now wanted to know how the immune system was dysregulated to result in TSS. I remember receiving my "pink sheet" review of my application. They were called pink sheets because indeed the reviews were printed on pink paper. All of us who received these sheets in the mail, as there was no internet at the time, went to the local bar, had a beer, and then had a friend open the envelope, fearing the worst. My pink sheet said: "Dr. Schlievert does not have sufficient expertise in immunology, biochemistry, and cell biology to perform the planned experiments." My thinking was that I was likely the only person with the expertise to perform such experiments. I thus called my National Institutes of Health Program officer who served as the interface between the anonymous grant review panel and investigator (me). My program officer, Dr. Milton Gordon (now deceased), told me that: "There is absolutely no interest at NIH in menstrual toxic shock syndrome." I was stunned. I pointed out to him that at least one-half of the United States—that is, at least women—were very concerned about the disease. He restated more emphatically: "Pat, there is absolutely no interest in toxic shock syndrome at NIH." Thus, I no longer had funding to study menstrual TSS. This was very disturbing to say the least. At that time, I did not know the reason for not funding my grant application, but I thought it was because this was a women's issue, and women's issues were *just not that important*. Now, I also believe it is because the CDC task force representatives convinced the grant review panel not to fund my continued research. After all, the CDC had solved the problem before the promised end of 1980, blaming the disease on Rely® tampons. I am sure now that both reasons are true.

There are other insidiously bad things that the CDC did in August-September 1980. They were very highly critical of the Tri-State TSS Study. I remember a meeting in Minnesota between the CDC and Tri-State TSS epidemiologists. The meeting was so explosively vitriolic that it is fortunate that no one had guns; some folks might not have survived the meeting. Clearly, the CDC did not believe that all tampons with risk going up as absorbency increased were associated. It was not until 1989 that the CDC finally agreed with the Tri-State epidemiologists. Even then they chose not to cite the 1982 Tri-State Study results.

Just as bad, some higher-up administrative individuals at the CDC called each of the major journals that publish on health issues, including menstrual TSS. The CDC wanted to be informed of all manuscripts and to be the reviewers of all manuscripts submitted for publication, in the name of "national security interest." I can only assume they wanted to review and reject manuscripts to prevent other tampons from being associated with menstrual TSS, so the promise to Senator Kennedy could become reality.

I already mentioned that I got nowhere stating to the CDC that there was another form of TSS, namely streptococcal TSS. It was not until I again publicized this new disease in 1987 that the CDC was dragged into recognizing streptococcal TSS. I should note that a researcher at the CDC (now deceased) said to me: "Pat, we simply did not see streptococcal syndrome as a problem, and as you say we were dragged in to investigate it." Indeed, streptococcal TSS was and is both more common than staphylococcal TSS, and its fatality rate when described was 85 percent. Half of the survivors have limbs amputated or major tissue parts of their bodies removed due to what is called necrotizing fasciitis and myositis. The term necrotizing is pretty self-explanatory. Fasciitis refers to infection along tissue planes, for example under the skin and spreading laterally. Myositis refers to infection of the muscles; necrotizing myositis at the time of first disease description was greater than 95 percent fatal. This disease is often referred to as the "flesh-eating disease".

The Deputy Chief of the CDC TSS task force, Dr. Bruce Dan (now deceased), testified in a supposed menstrual TSS case against a tampon manufacturer in San Jose, California. It has always been my impression that the CDC does not allow its public officials to testify in court cases; they are supposed to remain impartial. Be that as it may, Dr. Dan stated that TSS is associated with and caused by tampons, and that: "It does not matter if *Staphylococcus aureus* or Group A streptococcus is isolated. The disease is clinically defined, and the disease is associated with tampon use." The plaintiff won her case; please see https://law.justia.com/cases/california/court-of-appeal/3d/174/831.html. This case is important since *Staphylococcus aureus* was not isolated from the woman, despite hospital attempts to culture the bacteria. However, Group A streptococci were isolated from her throat. The woman was correctly treated with penicillin for her streptococcal infection, a treatment that would not treat staphylococcal TSS. Incidentally, she did not have Group A streptococci isolated vaginally. As I have stated, the reason for the tampon association with menstrual TSS is the introduction of oxygen (air) vaginally, required for production of TSS Toxin by *Staphylococcus aureus*. Group A streptococci function completely independently of oxygen in that their metabolism is that of an anaerobe (no air) and not an aerobe; we call them aerotolerant anaerobes. Thus, there is no way that any tampon use would influence production of scarlet fever toxin A. Plenty of this toxin was produced in the throat of the patient to cause her disease. Streptococcal TSS in women often occurs in association with menstrual periods, having nothing to do with tampon use. This is the reason I restate that menstrual refers only to the time of menstruation, but it does not state where the causative bacteria are isolated or which of the two types of bacteria (*Staphylococcus aureus* or Group A streptococci) caused the disease.

Thus, this case demonstrated a critically important problem. Opinions in a court of law do not necessarily agree with the science. This is by-and-large a problem of scientists both living in ivory towers and choosing not to get involved in cases, and not allowing the science as explained to juries to be believed. What I mean by the last part of the statement is that who does the jury believe, Dr. Dan representing the federal CDC, or me, the scientist at "only a public university", even if I was the reason we know so much about TSS? Clearly, the jury chose to believe Dr. Dan, even though he was dead wrong. As I stated above, he was not an expert on either *Staphylococcus aureus* or Group A streptococci, yet he was giving expert opinions. I asked a judge: "Do scientific witnesses NOT have to tell the truth anymore?"

He knew where I was going with this comment, and he replied: "The courts give expert scientific witnesses more leeway than is given to other witnesses."

If you find the things done by the CDC troubling, I think you should also consider a few other things. It is well recognized that the CDC did a "poor" job of investigating another disease that increased in incidence at the same time as menstrual TSS. When first identified, this other disease was called GRID, for Gay-Related Immune Deficiency. We now know this as HIV/AIDS. There is a book published entitled *And The Band Played On: Politics, People, and the Aids Epidemic* by Randy Shilts where the "screw-ups" of the CDC are emphasized.[43] I also note that there is a disease called Brainerd Diarrhea, named after an outbreak of long-lasting diarrhea in Brainerd, Minnesota, associated with drinking unpasteurized milk. Two years after the CDC "messed up" the epidemiology of this disease, I was asked to help solve what was causing the outbreak. I was not able to help because of the long duration since the beginning. I should note that even today I do not think we know the cause of Brainerd Diarrhea. We do know it is found in other parts of the United States in association with unpasteurized milk. I could go on for some time, but I want to give one other short example.

A physician friend of mine called me one day with a patient with recurrent menstrual TSS. The case was caused by a methicillin-resistant *Staphylococcus aureus* (MRSA). He wanted advice. I said to him: "The CDC would say…"

However, he cut me off with the comment: "We know the CDC could never give the proper advice, so I want you to tell me what to do."

I gave my standard answer: "Give vancomycin since the cause is an MRSA.

Give clindamycin to shut off TSS Toxin production. Give rifampin because of its mucosal surface penetrating ability. And, give intravenous immunoglobulin to neutralize TSS Toxin that was already present." The patient survived and has not had additional recurrences.

Overall, I think things have improved at the CDC since the 1980s. However, I worry. We know they have increased responsibilities, now called CDC and Prevention. We also know they have been short-shrifted in funding for years. We now see them having to handle the nationwide coronavirus infection. They already have messed up the COVID-19 testing, delaying the United States by 4-6 weeks by making a kit that did not work. They simply could have adopted the test that South Korea had already developed. I can only assume this lack of adopting an already developed test was part of the well-known CDC arrogance. They usually think they can do better than others, even if that is not true. It now appears that their role in COVID-19 has been marginalized in favor of Dr. Anthony Fauci of NIH's NIAID leading the national effort.

Chapter 9

September 1980 through 1983: I Can Clear a Restaurant in No Time: Why Tampons are Associated With Menstrual Toxic Shock Syndrome

A lot happened in 1980 through 1984 related to staphylococcal menstrual, vaginal TSS. Among these, many opinions largely based on no evidence were put forward to explain why tampons were associated with menstrual toxic shock syndrome. These discussions are the reasons I can clear restaurants in no time. Some folks even call me the tampon man. At this time, it also finally became recognized that non-menstrual TSS occurs.

Guys can become quite squeamish when it comes to tampons and menstruation. I can sit in restaurants or bars, speaking about cases with a group of scientists, and in no time, no one wants to sit anywhere near us. This happened many times, so it confirms my thinking that this continues to be taboo. I can appreciate this may turn folks off in restaurants, but bars? Come on. People speak about all kinds of things in bars.

I quote Laurie Garrett in her book *The Coming Plague*: "Feminine Hygiene is studied mostly by men."[44] Yes, that's the way it was back then and continues to be so even today. My entire career has been devoted to studies of women's health issues and microbes that affect their health. When I was a graduate student in microbiology and immunology at the University of Iowa from 1973-1976, I studied why human amniotic fluid is antimicrobial.[45] This is important, as it protects the developing fetus from infection. We identified a simple factor of six amino acids plus the metal zinc that protected the developing fetus. It is interesting to me that the peptide required the amino acid lysine. This was about the time Nobel Laureate Norman Borlaug developed high-lysine corn. Both lysine and zinc were deficient in developing countries. I remember the World Health Organization asking my mentor Dr. Rudy Galask how to reduce intrauterine deaths in developing countries. The answer became: Have pregnant women eat high-lysine corn, and have the women take zinc supplements. Many years later, an independent researcher called me and said: "Pat, that was the first defensin to be described." He wanted to know if I was still studying the factor. By then, I had moved on to menstrual TSS. It was more than ten years after receiving my PhD that the name defensin was coined for this family of antibacterial factors common in human fluids, including amniotic fluid.

The major question that had been asked since the beginning of the menstrual TSS epidemic was: "Why are tampons associated with menstrual, vaginal TSS?" I was the only researcher in the world at that time who had what we call hyperimmune antibodies against TSS Toxin available for my use in determining why tampons were associated. I had vaccinated a series of rabbits against TSS Toxin, making them hyperimmune. Like humans, not all rabbits could be vaccinated against the active toxin but 50 percent could. The remaining 50 percent ultimately died of TSS. Thus, I had a pool of antibodies that were very specific for reaction only to TSS Toxin. I also had diagnostic assays that I could use in my laboratory to tell how much TSS Toxin was being produced by menstrual TSS *Staphylococcus aureus*. These assays were both very specific and exceptionally sensitive. It is these same assays that allowed me to serve as a reference laboratory for the California laboratory doing TSS Toxin testing. Also, this is the reason so many physicians asked me to consult with them. I could tell if their patient did indeed have TSS by assessing if the isolated *Staphylococcus aureus* produced TSS Toxin. Remember, there are many variant forms of TSS that resemble other diseases. It is important to rule in or rule out TSS as the cause of the patient's illness. I could do this, and as I said I have consulted on over eight thousand cases of staphylococcal TSS.

Before I tell you "my story" of identification of the real reason for the tampon association with menstrual, vaginal TSS, namely introduction of oxygen (air) trapped within tampons, let me tell you a lot of opinions put forward to the news media without a shred of scientific data and which were invariably incorrect. I have come to say very cynically: "Let's never, ever let opinions of scientists be contaminated with scientific data to support their unfounded opinions." This continues even today in the TSS field. I also remember the poem "The Microbe" by Hilaire Belloc (deceased) in which the last two lines are: "Oh! Let us never, never doubt what nobody is sure about." This poem is in the public domain and can be read at http://www.yourdailypoem.com/listpoem.jsp?poem_id=1469.

You will notice that I said *tampon association with TSS* and not *tampon cause of TSS*. Very early on in the menstrual TSS story, there were many folks with marginal understanding of TSS who thought tampons, such as Rely® brand tampons, caused TSS. I remember one group of researchers who developed a model of menstrual TSS in of all things chickens. They cut up pieces of tampons and placed them in the uteruses of chickens. The chickens very quickly developed a disease in which their combs turned blue, and they died. There was never any evidence of other symptoms, and TSS *Staphylococcus aureus* were never isolated from the chickens. Additionally, women do not place tampons in their uteruses. I am not sure what disease the chickens were suffering from, except maybe extreme trauma, but they did not have menstrual TSS. We know with 100 percent certainty that menstrual, vaginal staphylococcal TSS is caused by TSS Toxin-producing *Staphylococcus aureus*.

When I was a faculty member at UCLA in the summer of 1980, after I started the major publicity on toxic shock syndrome, I saw a question and answer meeting on TSS that was being held at the Women's Center at UCLA. It was open to the public. I went to the meeting, and I was NOT surprised that I was the only male in attendance. Maybe this was again "squeamish male syndrome". An undergraduate student in the audience asked a question to the moderators as to why tampons caused TSS. She had seen that someone had written on the wall of the women's locker room at UCLA: "Rely Kills!" The answer given surprised me, and the answer was that the disease was caused by Rely® tampons, which had a different construction than other tampons (teabag versus tube design), implying that tampon composition and construction caused the disease. This discussion went on for nearly thirty minutes, and at that time I stepped in and raised the following point. I said that the bacterium *Staphylococcus aureus* is the cause, not tampons, and all high-absorbency tampons are co-causally linked to the disease. This was unsettling to the group needless to say. The moderators asked: "Well who are you to think you know anything about this subject? It is a women's issue." I then told them that I was in fact the person who started the publicity on the disease so women would know there was indeed a disease that was caused by TSS Toxin (then called PE C) -producing *Staphylococcus aureus*. Also, I noted that Dr. Shirley Fannin, LA County Health Department, and I had already noted that the CDC was wrong to blame menstrual TSS solely on use of Rely® tampons, as all high-absorbency tampons were associated in proportion equal to their commercial sales numbers. I then joined the moderators in the discussion. In the end, this was a terrific meeting, and it showed how willing young women were to learn about their health... even if it was from a "tampon" guy.

Later in the news media, newspapers, radio, and television, again without data, many biomedical scientists were asked by reporters why tampons caused menstrual TSS. They should have answered: "Tampons alone do not cause TSS, but we do not know why they are associated." Instead, they had many half-baked opinions. I will give you some. Yes, I am being a bit snarky, but I think I am justified, as you will see in the next several paragraphs.

I remember one very well-placed physician espousing: "Tampons form a vaginal plug, which creates a vaginal environment devoid of oxygen (anaerobic), and together these two things allow the staphylococcal bacteria to make the causative toxin."

The same news reporter called me and asked my thought on this "pretty cool" theory. My response was adamant: "No way! That statement is not true, and it will not be true even if spoken in a louder voice. It would be nice if that biomedical scientist would contaminate his opinions with data." The reporter published the theory anyway. After all, the well-placed physician with no data was certainly more knowledgeable than that young PhD upstart at UCLA who started the publicity to make the American public aware of the disease. And to think, I told the reporter why that theory was incorrect, and I also told him what the real reason was for the tampon association. Here is what I said: "Tampons leak, and thus they do not form plugs. Any woman can tell you that." Even today, I know of young women who participate in sports and do not want spotting, so dangerously to their health use two tampons at a time. Likewise, I said: "TSS Toxin (then called PE C) requires oxygen (air) for it to be produced, the opposite of an environment without oxygen." So… the physician was wrong for two of two reasons. By the way, the reason it is dangerous for young women to use two tampons today is that this effectively increases absorbency vaginally, approaching the absorbency levels of the high-absorbency tampons marketed up until 1984. This introduces a lot of oxygen vaginally, allowing a lot of TSS Toxin to be produced, and putting the young women at risk. I agree with the current CDC and FDA recommendations: "If you choose to use tampons, use the lowest absorbency tampons to control menstrual flow. Do not use any tampon beyond eight hours."

Another research group from large East Coast universities wanted to explain why Rely® tampons were "the only causes". They stated: "Rely® tampons contain chips" of what Procter & Gamble called CLD for cross-linked derivative of the molecule carboxy-methyl cellulose. Don't you just love those chemical terms? Anyway, this research group simply knew that CLD is broken down to the sugar glucose by other bacteria in the vaginas of women. The bacteria *Staphylococcus aureus* then use glucose as a food source to produce TSS Toxin.[46] For a short period of time, the CDC bought into this, even publishing a manuscript on the subject; they rightly so never pursued this further. This theory was again reported in newspapers and on radio and TV as true. However, the theory is dead wrong for four of four reasons.

First, women simply do not have bacteria vaginally that degrade carboxy-methyl cellulose. Women are not like sheep and cows that graze on grass, taking in cellulose in grass, and degrading the cellulose to glucose. Indeed, at a much later date, a relatively obnoxious researcher friend of mine noted that: "No woman has inserted a tampon and pulled out only a string with the tampon degraded." He was cynically noting that some other tube-variety tampons contained carboxy-methyl cellulose, and if women had vaginal microbes that degraded this molecule, then the women would pull out only a string.

Second, glucose suppresses production of TSS Toxin by *Staphylococcus aureus*.[15] Think about it this way: If you have all the nice sugar in the world to grow, why would you want to make a poison that can kill women? *Staphylococcus aureus* only makes TSS Toxin when it becomes threatened by a lack of glucose; it sees this lack of glucose as a danger signal for "I need more food". I showed this conclusively and published my findings in February 1983 *Journal of Infectious Diseases* as cited just at the start of this paragraph.

Third, this research group also said Rely® tampons were causal because contact with menstrual blood turned the tampons into an emulsion; emulsions are unique in that they lead to the bacteria producing TSS Toxin. Think of emulsion as meringue. Meringue is made by vigorous mixing of eggs and sugar—that is, mixing in lots and lots of air. They did not realize that emulsion was a surrogate for air. They thought this was independent of my study already published which I will mention in detail for the role of oxygen in later paragraphs.

Finally and fourth, my cynical scientist friend was correct for another reason. Yes, other tampons contained carboxy-methyl cellulose, but in fact some of them were of such low absorbency, they were never associated with menstrual TSS. If carboxy-methyl cellulose degradation was so important, why was it not important in those low absorbency tampons not associated with TSS? Thus and collectively, this theory by this research group did not hold any water, not then and not even today, though they continue to espouse it as true. Why did they get so much play in the news media? They were at large East Coast private universities, and clearly they were more knowledgeable than I was.

When I was at UCLA, I was approached by the producer of a TV show *Quincy, M.E.* as played by Jack Klugman. The producer asked me to help them come up with a scenario in which Dr. Quincy could solve the menstrual TSS tampon problem. The producer wanted Dr. Quincy to discover that tampon manufacturers, notable Procter & Gamble who made Rely® tampons, were adding arsenic to tampons to increase menstrual bleeding, which in turn would lead to more menstrual, vaginal toxic shock syndrome. This thinking for some reason caught on for a while as a thought for why tampons "caused" TSS. There is absolutely no evidence for any such addition of arsenic to tampons. I will note, however, that maybe this theory came up because nearly all menstrual toxic shock syndrome *Staphylococcus aureus* are resistant to both cadmium and arsenic. Although this is true, arsenic is never added to tampons to increase menstrual blood flow. It is also possible that women were coming to realize that there were additives in some tampons, so maybe arsenic was also added to increase menstrual bleeding. I say again: "This simply is not now and never, ever has been true".

I would like to have a short aside for a few minutes. I had a phone conversation with my long-time collaborator where I suggested that we look at the genetic DNA element that was controlling TSS Toxin production. He said to me: "That is not important." I thought it was important since cadmium and arsenic resistance, combined with penicillin resistance, are usually controlled by plasmid mobile genetic elements of DNA. That is not the case with cadmium, arsenic, and penicillin resistance in TSS *Staphylococcus aureus*, since most strains lack plasmids. Additionally, in that phone call I thought we should try to find out what controlled that production of TSS Toxin, and if it was linked in any way to cadmium, arsenic, and penicillin resistance. Imagine my surprise when a year later my collaborator, without me, published that TSS Toxin was on a pathogenicity island of DNA in the bacteria.[47] This was the first such island found in *Staphylococcus aureus*.

My friend Dr. Gregory Bohach, a former postdoctoral associate of mine, called me and said: "I'll bet that makes you angry." He knew that I had called my collaborator previously where the collaborator said this project was of insufficient interest to pursue scientifically.

Back on track: I'd like to tell you the story of a menstrual toxic shock syndrome trial case in Wisconsin in which I participated. This case involved Tampax® Super and occurred prior to when uniform standards of tampon absorbency were put in place. Tampax® Super sounds like a high-absorbency tampon doesn't it? However, as I mentioned the TSS case occurred in the early 1980s, prior to uniform labeling standards. This tampon was in fact the second lowest absorbency tampon on the market. The Tri-State Epidemiology Study, the gold standard, did not find an association with the tampon.[5] The reason this case is so interesting is because the trial showed something important about some biomedical scientists and their "bad" opinions. The defense attorney in this trial was Mr. Roger Podesta, Debevoise and Plimpton, New York. The plaintiff's case, as stated by the plaintiff attorney, depended to a large extent on the testimony of a scientist who was the microscopist in a study of tampons and their possible cause of micro-ulcerations vaginally.[48] As stated by the microscopist, these micro-ulcerations of vaginal mucosa would lead to increased TSS Toxin production in those micro-ulcerations and greater TSS Toxin access to the body. The microscopist was called to testify on behalf of the plaintiff in the case. He went through his testimony stating that Tampax® Super tampons were indeed high absorbency because of their name, and were thus associated with menstrual TSS because of micro-ulcerations caused by the tampon. He did not know that Tampax® Super tampon was actually the second lowest absorbency tampon on the market. He said that the micro-ulcerations produced then allowed TSS *Staphylococcus aureus* to grow and make TSS Toxin, which would easily gain access to the bloodstream. After his direct examination, the most amazing cross-examination took place. The cross-examination was by Mr. Podesta. He first completely took the witness through the direct examination again to make it fresh in the minds of the jurors. This included the statement that Tampax® Super was high absorbency, caused vaginal micro-ulcerations, and led to TSS Toxin production vaginally with increased penetration of the TSS Toxin into the bloodstream, again because of the micro-ulcerations. Mr. Podesta then provided a letter to the witness from Mr. Robert Underhill, then Vice President for Research for Kimberly Clark. It turns out that Kimberly Clark funded the study on vaginal micro-ulcerations, to which the microscopist was referring. The microscopist was asked to read the letter. It turns out that the low absorbency tampon, which DID NOT cause vaginal micro-ulcerations was Tampax® Super, the tampon that was the basis for the lawsuit. It is also important to state that TSS Toxin, once produced vaginally by *Staphylococcus aureus*, does not need micro-ulcerations to gain access to the bloodstream. It easily, on its own power, makes its way into the blood.

I learned some things from this lawsuit: 1) As a scientist, do not overstate what you know. In this case, the plaintiff's main witness was a microscopist who did not know of the Kimberly Clark letter explaining which tampons were low versus high absorbency (there was another team member who did know, but he was deceased and the letter was never available ahead of time for the microscopist); 2) I watched and was amazed by Mr. Podesta. He would be my lawyer of choice if I needed one in such a case. I did notice, however, that his pant-leg was shaking while doing the examination of the plaintiff witness, indicating he has nerves just like the rest of us; 3) And most importantly, vaginal micro-ulcerations do not explain the tampon association with menstrual TSS.

Now my studies on the reason for the tampon association: After months of answering questions about tampon roles, I pointed out that they must be bringing something into the vagina that stimulated TSS Toxin production by *Staphylococcus aureus*. This must be true since all high-absorbency tampons were associated, so it could not be their composition and construction. Risk of menstrual TSS was associated with absorbency, with risk going up with increased absorbency. In 1981, I did an analysis of what factors would promote TSS Toxin production, taking a very broad approach. Remember, I had the ability to quantify TSS Toxin production in my laboratory because I had those highly specific hyperimmune antibodies from rabbits.

I showed first that TSS Toxin production depended on protein, not sugar, being present as a food source. My observations on why tampons are associated with menstrual TSS are all published in.[15] As I noted above, when I added glucose, TSS Toxin production was actually suppressed. This makes sense since there are lots of proteins present vaginally during menstruation, and they are broken down to amino acids required for synthesis of the toxin, which in turn is made up of linked amino acids, now in a toxic arrangement.

I then also showed that body temperature (98.6°F) was needed for excellent TSS Toxin production by *Staphylococcus aureus*, with lower temperatures not favoring toxin production, and higher temperature, including 104°F, stimulating TSS Toxin production. Like proteins, the correct body temperature was present in the vagina during menstruation.

Next, I showed that pH (acidic versus basic) was important. Acidic pH, like present vaginally at times other than menstruation, both prevented *Staphylococcus aureus* growth and inhibited production of TSS Toxin. Neutral pH near 7, as would be present during menstruation, was required for *Staphylococcus aureus* growth and TSS Toxin production. Earlier in this book I mentioned to you that only during menstruation do *Staphylococcus aureus* grow vaginally, and at that time they grow up into the billions. They completely take over the vaginal microbiome by day two to three of menstruation, a time when they can produce a lot of TSS Toxin.

In all of these studies, the only thing that did not fit with tampon use and risk of TSS was that I showed that oxygen (air) was required for TSS Toxin production, and that the vagina in the absence of high-absorbency tampons was without oxygen. This was both simple and it meshed with all of the known epidemiology perfectly: As women use tampons, they introduce air (oxygen) into an environment that normally lacks oxygen. The amount of oxygen is a function of absorbency with larger tampons introducing more oxygen. Oxygen was absolutely required for TSS Toxin production even though it was not required for *Staphylococcus aureus* growth vaginally. This microbe can grow in the absence and presence of oxygen, but it can only make TSS Toxin when oxygen is present. Later, my laboratory identified the gene regulatory mechanism that is required to control the oxygen effect.[49] That bacterial regulatory system shuts off TSS Toxin production in the absence of oxygen and allows TSS Toxin to be produced when oxygen is present.

It is indeed interesting to me how my experimentation ultimately overcame opinions. I published this high-profile manuscript in February 1983 in the *Journal of Infectious Diseases*,[15] the journal that became the sounding board on menstrual TSS. However, the struggle was not over. Even in that publication, the reviewers who advised the editor of the journal on publication worthiness did not allow me to say oxygen was the reason for the tampon association. They only allowed me to say: "Somehow the vagina becomes oxygenated in the presence of high-absorbency tampons."

I want to call this next section "a whole lotta nothing". There have been research groups that continually, even today, suggest that the tampon association is because of unnatural components of tampons or not because of oxygen introduction within tampons. One group has advocated the use of "all cotton" tampons, which they state do not allow TSS Toxin production, in contrast to TSS Toxin production in rayon cotton blend and all rayon tampons. None of the rest of the research community has been able to verify their findings, despite four research groups trying to verify them.

I have said earlier many times in this book that the major association of tampons with menstrual TSS risk is because of oxygen introduction within tampons. I have been called by many news sources, and I participated in many additional studies related to oxygen and "unnatural components" in tampons. Let me first quell the naysayers in regards to oxygen.

There was an investigator from Leeds, England, who made a strong comment at a menstrual TSS Symposium in which he stated: "I can think of a way that TSS Toxin can be produced in the absence of oxygen. Dr. Schlievert is wrong in saying oxygen is absolutely required for TSS Toxin production." This stunned me since just immediately before him I had given a presentation showing that oxygen was absolutely required. When asked, however, this other investigator refused to reveal how TSS Toxin could be produced in the absence of oxygen. The overall reason for his statement, however, was for the research community present to think: "Dr. Schlievert does not know what he is talking about, thinking oxygen is the explanation. Again, he's just a Midwestern dumbshit!" That evening at dinner and after that other investigator had had a few too many drinks, he explained to me and adjacent diners how this could happen—that is, to get TSS Toxin production in the absence of oxygen. I forced his hand to have him repeat this conversation in front of the very same symposium audience the next day so I could make a key point. Here was his presentation: "You take toxic shock syndrome *Staphylococcus aureus* and adhere them to a screen with very tiny holes in it. Oxygen can pass through the holes, but *Staphylococcus aureus* cannot. Then, you remove the oxygen from the medium on the side containing the *Staphylococcus aureus*. Thus, the bacteria are without oxygen. Then, and this is the key part, you pass oxygen by on the opposing side of the bacteria adhered to the screen. They gain oxygen from that other side to make TSS Toxin, but the medium they are in continues to be without oxygen." This points out important things. Oxygen is in fact being supplied to the bacteria, and it is absolutely required for TSS Toxin production. Scientists, if that is what you can call such a person, must be called-out when they make outrageous, and idiotic even, statements such as "oxygen is not required for TSS Toxin production", when they lack even remotely appropriate data to support their claim. I remember the amazing experiments being done by a graduate student of mine, now Dr. Jeremy Yarwood. When we were studying the oxygen effect on TSS Toxin production, one day Jeremy pumped oxygen into our apparatus just as fast as he could. The bacteria at high cell density, however, were using the oxygen so fast that the medium remained devoid of oxygen, and the oxygen flow was so fast it caused the apparatus to freeze, stopping everything. I came to appreciate that *Staphylococcus aureus* heavily uses all available oxygen to produce TSS Toxin.

In the autumn of 1982, my friend Dr. Sydney Finegold (deceased) asked me to give the Presidential Address at the Infectious Diseases Society of America on what I knew about menstrual, vaginal TSS. He was then the president of the society. It is important to mention that he "asked" me to do this, and that I did not in some way coerce him into asking me, as if I could do such a thing. This will become important in a few paragraphs. There were nearly 1700 infectious diseases physicians in the audience. Wow!

I gave the presentation, and two things that are important to me happened as a result. First, I had been in constant communication with my friend Dr. Michael Osterholm, Head of the Tri-State TSS task force. In more than one of these conversations, we had discussed why tampons were associated with TSS as a function of absorbency. I had told him that all of my data said that oxygen introduction vaginally was the key. At the end of my presentation, Mike was the first to ask a question: "Pat, you and I have had many conversations, so why don't you tell everyone why tampons are associated with menstrual TSS?" I explained the oxygen theory that I published in the subsequent February 1983 *Journal of Infectious Diseases*. Nearly everyone agreed with me as I look back on it, which was nice to see. However...

There was one infectious diseases physician in attendance who thought I, as a young researcher, was making established investigators "look bad" by collecting so much data in such a short period of time. This physician scientist was the head of an infectious diseases division at a major university. It turns out he had spoken with friends of mine the day prior to my presentation, telling them he was angry and that he was going to give me a bad time for, as I said, making too much progress in such a short period of time. He did not know these infectious diseases researchers were friends of mine. My friends told me of his plans. These are truly the kinds of friends I need and value! After my presentation, this physician did indeed try to cause trouble by standing up and saying: "You have gone so fast in your work that you have not even considered some very important things, such as the important role of the metal iron in production of TSS Toxin. You should have gone slower in your investigations to present a more credible story." I knew something was going to happen, but I did not know exactly what was going to happen. However, it is always my policy to give credit to all of my colleagues in presentations. After my speech, I thanked and acknowledged the contributions of an enormous number of infectious diseases physicians, so he was attacking them as well as me. However, I knew the answer to his comment. I had in fact considered the possible role of iron. I asked the slide projector person to return to a slide. On that slide, I presented data that I did not discuss, because it was unimportant data. Iron had no role in TSS Toxin production. The questioner sputtered a few seconds and then sat down. Remember, Sydney asked me to give this presentation. I did not in some way coerce him into having me do it.

My collaborators and I have now verified the requirement of oxygen vaginally in women. The same conditions must be met that I found in my February 1983 article in the *Journal of Infectious Diseases.*

I want to return only briefly to the discussion of "all natural" cotton tampons versus other kinds of tampons, namely those made of cotton and rayon blend and those made of all rayon. First, it is important to recognize that cotton and rayon are essentially the same thing. Cotton comes from cotton plants, whereas rayon comes from trees. However, they contain the same chemical components. Second, if you examine tampons, you will notice that the fibers can be worked into tube shapes. Most cotton and rayon that I have seen are "fly-away" materials, kind of like dandelions that have gone to seed. Most if not all tampons have what are called surfactants to keep this "fly-away" effect under control. These compounds either have no effect on production of TSS Toxin or interfere with its production.

There is a research group who have published that "all cotton" tampons do not allow TSS Toxin production, and any small amount that is produced is trapped by the ability of cotton to bind irreversibly to the TSS Toxin.[50] Research groups have disputed those findings and published to the effect that they disagree.[515253] Some were studies where the researchers were blinded as to the tampon brand being tested. In all cases, there was no difference between "all cotton" and other compositions of tampons.

The Canadian Broadcasting Company spoke with me about this "great all cotton theory", knowing that "all natural" is better sounding than other fibers. Most folks do not appreciate that rayon is natural, but its name sounds like nylon which is synthetic. I thus performed a blinded study with the Canadian Broadcasting Company, where I did not know the tampon varieties being tested. When the study was unblinded, as I expected, there was no difference between the kinds of fibers in the tampons and TSS Toxin production. The theory pops up even occasionally today that "all cotton" tampons are somehow better than cotton-rayon blend or all rayon tampons. The theory is easily dispelled.

It can be dangerous for women to think they are safe from menstrual toxic shock syndrome if they use "all cotton" tampons. Cotton tampons, like other kinds of tampons, come in regular, super, and super plus varieties. Risk of TSS increases with increased absorbency, just like with tampons that are not all cotton. The only difference is if women buy into the argument that "all cotton" tampons are somehow safer… which they are not.

This does raise a critical topic however. Because of the shift of the United States population to value the use of "all natural" products in general, this has also penetrated the tampon industry. Soon after Rely® tampons were removed from the market, some women shifted to the use of sea sponges as "natural" alternatives to tampons. What do sponges look like? Bags of air is what they look like to me. I even have a photograph of me scuba diving in the Caribbean inside of a very large sponge. You get the message, I hope. These sponges were also associated with menstrual TSS. However, there is an even more important message. Since these were natural products, they also contained other natural things found in the ocean. Women developed strong allergies to many of the dead sea creatures that had been living inside the sponges.

I recently was asked to comment on whether it is okay in emergency situations to use a cosmetic sponge to control menstrual flow. I said: "Yes, in emergency situations, it is likely to be okay. Just don't do this repetitively."

In the *Journal of Infectious Diseases* (March 1983), I published the summary of my presentation at the Infectious Diseases Society of America meeting.[31] To briefly summarize:

I said TSS Toxin (still called PE C) was the cause.

I gave a model for how TSS Toxin causes the disease, a model that remains correct today.

I stated why tampons were associated with menstrual TSS, the only reason that has withstood the test of time.

I explained why 20 percent of women do not develop antibodies to protect themselves from menstrual TSS.

This has become a very high-profile paper, and the findings are as true today as they were way back then.

There are many other things that happened shortly after Rely® tampons were removed from the market, things that merit discussion.

The CDC wished to know from where *Staphylococcus aureus* producing TSS Toxin came. At this time the name of the toxin had not been decided upon, but I will use it for ease of presentation. The CDC hypothesized that women at tampon manufacturing plants were contaminating equipment and tampon component parts, such that then the final tampons were contaminated. The CDC threatened to close down tampon manufacturing plants. This hypothesis seemed highly unlikely to me and to my friend Michael Osterholm, Minnesota State Epidemiologist at the time. Mike and I were asked to present to the CDC our observations that related to their thoughts on this theory. Thus, on Easter weekend in 1982, Mike and I flew to the CDC in Atlanta. Interestingly, we flew on Northwest Airlines (now Delta), and there were only five passengers on the plane that held more than two hundred. The airline moved all of us to first class.

The next day, Monday, I presented to the CDC that 5-10 percent of all women across the United States at any given time have TSS Toxin *Staphylococcus aureus* vaginally, whether or not they use tampons. Thus, there was no need to invoke the thought that women working in tampon manufacturing plants were contaminating tampons. Additionally, I have been at many of such plants to observe their operation. There is virtually no human contact with tampon manufacturing. Finally, I had cultured many thousands of unused tampons, and I never found one contaminated with *Staphylococcus aureus*, even though they are not sold as sterile.

I performed another very interesting study related to where the TSS Toxin *Staphylococcus aureus* came from related to menstrual TSS. Dr Bill Altemeier (now deceased) had collected *Staphylococcus aureus* as vaginal cultures from women since the 1940s. He sent me, in blinded fashion, strains from 1940 through 1981. I tested them one at a time for ability to produce TSS Toxin. There were as many as one hundred tested for each year. What did I find when the code was broken? TSS Toxin-positive *Staphylococcus aureus* was present in the US even in 1940, but it was present in only very low numbers. The strain emerged in 1972 as a dominant microbe on mucosal surfaces.[4]

Recently, an undergraduate and graduate student in my laboratory together showed that a *Staphylococcus aureus* strain from Bundaberg, Australia produced TSS Toxin.[27] This strain was isolated in 1928 from a disaster in which twelve of twenty-four children who were administered antibodies to diphtheria toxin died due to contamination with this *Staphylococcus aureus*. Thus, these children died of TSS.

The TSS Toxin was present in *Staphylococcus aureus* strains all the way back to 1928. This then begs the question: Did the use of very high-absorbency tampons cause an emergence of TSS Toxin-producing bacteria? Alternatively, was it a coincidence? Bill Altemeier and I showed that the TSS Toxin-positive bacteria, although present in very low numbers before 1970, actually emerged in 1972 to become the dominant mucous membrane *Staphylococcus aureus* strain. Many physicians have said to me that if they saw a case of menstrual TSS, the disease occurred after 1972. They saw cases, but they just did not know what they were. This TSS Toxin-positive strain of *Staphylococcus aureus* peaked in occurrences in 1975, but it rose rapidly after 1972. The very high-absorbency tampons were introduced into the market in 1976. Thus, the emergence happened in 1972 independent of use of the highest absorbency tampons. In other words, this was an unfortunate coincidence.

The question still remains as to why the TSS Toxin-positive strain emerged in the first place. I have come to appreciate that *Staphylococcus aureus* strains emerge every ten years. This likely depends on how long it takes for the majority of the human population to develop immunity to the bacterium, such that when the majority of folks become immune, the strain dies back to a low level, only to reemerge later. I can cite multiple examples of this with other *Staphylococcus aureus* strains.

Staphylococcus aureus has long been recognized as a scourge in hospitals. The majority of current hospital cleanliness practices are in place to reduce *Staphylococcus aureus* infections. Even now, there are more than five hundred thousand surgical site infections in hospitals in the United States each year due to *Staphylococcus aureus*.

Let's look at *Staphylococcus aureus* infections across time in hospitals beginning in the 1950s. It is absolutely clear that in the early 1950s a strain called "29/52" emerged to peak in 1955 in hospitals, causing enormous numbers of serious infections, only to die back by 1960. However, a new variety of *Staphylococcus aureus* called "52/52A" came into hospitals in the early 1960s, peaking in 1965, causing large numbers of serious infections, only to die back in 1970. Then, we see the emergence of the TSS Toxin-positive strain in the 1970s. This strain emerged to peak in 1975, but for an unknown reason did not die back by 1980. The strain remains even today in fairly high percentages of humans colonized. The strain must have some selective advantage to allow it to persist in the face of the human immune system. My bet is that this strain of *Staphylococcus aureus* persists because TSS Toxin significantly prevents development of immunity by dysregulating the immune system.

In the 1990s, we saw the emergence of a strain of *Staphylococcus aureus* that was a bit different. It was what we call a methicillin-resistant *Staphylococcus aureus*, also known as MRSA. This strain was called USA400 and caused exceptionally serious and fatal infections, many in children, for about ten years, and then it also died back.

In the past ten years, we saw the emergence of a strain called USA300. This MRSA strain, in both the community and in hospitals, caused enormous numbers of extensive soft tissue infections (boils and abscesses). This organism caused infections in prisoners, pro-football players, wrestlers, and anyone else who had close contact with each other. The strain is now well on the way to dying back.

An unfortunate thing is that the scientific community is so focused on USA300, or whatever strain is currently emerging, that it is likely we will not know what new strain is emerging until the mid-2020s. This is unfortunate, but it is consistent with the majority of scientists wanting to protect their current work as the most important research. My thought, and I have been criticized for this thinking, is that we should focus on all of the major kinds of *Staphylococcus aureus*, and all at the same time. Additionally, we must come to recognize that *Staphylococcus aureus* strains that cause mucous membrane infections typically will be confined to mucous membranes. This is as opposed to strains that cause skin infections, where different factors are required for those strains to cause skin disease. For example, there is a toxin that kills human epithelial cells called alpha toxin that is responsible for the necrotic, damaged skin associated with boils. All strains of *Staphylococcus aureus* causing boils and other soft tissue infections on the skin produce this toxin in high amounts. Mucous membrane *Staphylococcus aureus* strains make very little if any of this toxin. In other words, alpha toxin is important for skin infections but not for strains on mucous membranes. This does not mean you cannot find mucous membrane strains on skin, but if you do, they will be present in damaged skin, such as surgical sites. *Staphylococcus aureus* is really the major bacterial type that can cause skin infections in the presence of normal, intact skin.

Let's go back to the CDC and their hypotheses. After we convinced the CDC not to shut down tampon production facilities, the CDC hypothesized that TSS Toxin production by *Staphylococcus aureus* came from the normal skin and mucous membrane bacteria, *Staphylococcus epidermidis*, through gene transfer from one species to another. It was thought that since this has happened occasionally with other genes in the past, it must be true here as well; in fact they thought it was very highly likely. I had already tested many *Staphylococcus epidermidis* bacteria for ability to make TSS Toxin, and I found none ever made the toxin.[54] This did not convince the CDC since I had not specifically tested strains that might be on unused tampons being sold to women. The CDC thus came to the Minneapolis-St. Paul, Minnesota area, a hot-spot for menstrual TSS, and bought up nearly all tampons on store shelves one weekend. They then asked the Food and Drug Administration employees in Minneapolis to isolate bacteria that might be on the tampons. I should add that folks told me that this amounted to many thousands of tampons being tested. The Food and Drug Administration folks found bacterial growth on twenty-two tampons. None of these were *Staphylococcus aureus*. However, the Food and Drug Administration found twenty-two *Staphylococcus epidermidis* strains. I do not know where those strains came from, other than what the readers should know, that even in hospitals, *Staphylococcus epidermidis* is often a contaminant coming from laboratory personnel handling the specimens along the way. But who knows where?

The important thing is that I tested all twenty-two strains for TSS Toxin in the usual way. I found none produced TSS Toxin, as I expected. I told this to the CDC TSS task force, and then I immediately went onto the CDC "shit list" for about a year. In the meantime, the CDC then asked Dr. Merlin Bergdoll to test the same microbes. He found that some of the twenty-two strains produced TSS Toxin.

Merlin was now considered a saint by the CDC. Remember that Merlin had previously published in *The Lancet* that some *Staphylococcus epidermidis* strains could make TSS Toxin.[28] This of course was later shown not to be true.

At about the same time, a friend of mine and Merlin's at Uniformed Services Medical Center, Dr. Matthew Pollack, had four *Staphylococcus aureus* strains that he said came from menstrual toxic shock syndrome patients. He asked both Merlin and me to test the strains for ability to produce TSS Toxin. I found all four strains were positive; Merlin found all four were negative. This caused lots of consternation obviously, so to resolve the issue, Merlin and I exchanged strains, with the thought there may have been a mix-up in sending strains to each of us that could explain our divergent findings. I again found that all four of the exchanged strains produced TSS Toxin, whereas Merlin found they were all negative. Hmmm!

Prior to reporting these discordant results to Matt Pollack, Merlin called me. He said: "Pat, I don't know what has happened, but my hyperimmune antibodies to TSS Toxin are not recognizing TSS Toxin; they are recognizing something else. I do not have the ability to tell what bacteria do and do not make TSS Toxin. Can you help me by providing some hyperimmune antibodies that you have?" Indeed, I did help Merlin, and from then on we always agreed on production of TSS Toxin.

We both informed Matt Pollack that indeed his strains made TSS Toxin. However, when Merlin went back to test the twenty-two *Staphylococcus epidermidis* strains from the CDC, like me, he found that all were negative for ability to produce TSS Toxin. Now, he too was on the CDC "shit list" as well as me. That hypothesis quickly went out the scientific window. I should note that no one, not a single person, has ever shown that any *Staphylococcus epidermidis* strain produces TSS Toxin. It is a shame that so many of us had to waste a lot of time on this theory when we could have been pursuing something more productive.

Menstrual toxic shock syndrome is unlike any other disease I know of. The Tri-State Toxic Shock Syndrome Study, published in the *Journal of Infectious Diseases* in 1982, showed that women who continue to use tampons, and even some women who do not, will develop recurrences of menstrual toxic shock syndrome.[5] I have had women call me after having six episodes asking that if they have a hysterectomy will this go away. I tell them there are easier things to do…

for example receive intravenous immunoglobulin. When they receive this treatment, they then have no more episodes. So, why do these recurrences happen? As shown by members of the Wisconsin Health Department and confirmed in a grand way by Dr. Jeffrey Parsonnet, there is a continual rise in percentages of folks developing antibodies to TSS Toxin with age.[10,30] At about three months of age, no infants have antibodies; prior to that they may have passively obtained antibodies from their moms during pregnancy, but they go away in three months. Thus, from three months of age until twelve years old there is a steady rise in persons who develop protective antibodies. There are three important points about this rise in antibodies. As many as 20 percent of women will never develop antibodies to TSS Toxin. No one knows what disease if any the 80 percent of children have that leads them to develop antibodies. Approximately twelve years of age is the time of onset of menstruation in girls today. I will discuss all three of these in a bit more detail.

We have ideas of why 20 percent of women, and I should also add men, do not develop antibodies. Women are of greater concern since they have menstrual periods that make them susceptible monthly to toxic shock syndrome. Men do not have these repetitive cycles and environments that allow toxic shock syndrome *Staphylococcus aureus* to grow and produce TSS Toxin. It turns out the immune system becomes so over-activated and produces so much interferon gamma that the ability to produce protective antibodies is lost in these folks. In the absence of antibodies, they can develop recurrences. Women who continue to use tampons have higher recurrence rates than women who discontinue use of tampons. However, even women who never again use tampons develop recurrences, just not to the extent as women who continue to use tampons. These women are also susceptible to post-influenza toxic shock syndrome caused by TSS Toxin. In children, my experience is that this is 100 percent fatal. Thus, all folks should get the influenza vaccine for as much protection as possible. I follow several families, and I can assure you this is a scary experience for their young daughters. It's like a time bomb waiting to go off each month during winter and spring months.

We simply do not know what disease if any the children develop in the twelve-year period of linear rise in antibodies. Dr. Chet Whitley and I tried to publish a manuscript describing toxic shock syndrome in infants. We were never able to do so because the reviewers said the infants did not have toxic shock syndrome. This made no sense to me. Infants often do not show fever, rash, and even hypotension. They are likely to become lethargic and show many of the multi-organ changes in toxic shock syndrome, but they will likely have two missing symptoms. When we tried to publish the paper, it had not yet been established that infants may not show all symptoms. I have said before the following saying: "Let us never doubt what no one is sure about." The biomedical community was so sure we were wrong, yet we were publishing in uncharted territory. It is a shame because this could have set the stage for finding out what the kids have. Japanese researchers have now extensively described TSS in young children, just not the United States. What were we thinking?

The third point I made above is that menstrual periods are beginning in eleven to twelve-year-olds rather than twelve to fifteen-year-olds these days. Menstrual periods are quite irregular early in their onset. There are then several things that influence use of tampons in these twelve-year-olds. It used to be that menstrual TSS occurred primarily in fifteen to twenty-one-year-olds. Now we see the major incidence in eleven to fourteen-year-olds. We have shown that these young girls/women have menstrual periods with minimal blood flow but lots of vaginal secretions. Our studies show that this favors TSS Toxin production. Blood actually reduces TSS Toxin production. In other words, the parts of used tampons where you find TSS Toxin are the parts where there are vaginal secretions and little if any blood. Anthropomorphically speaking, *Staphylococcus aureus* does not like to be in the presence of blood; the organism very quickly walls itself off from blood and additionally the immune system. This is clearly a survival advantage to the microbe. In my speaking with young girls/women, they are likely to be highly active in sports or activities where menstrual spotting would be highly embarrassing. Thus, they may use two tampons at a time, greatly increasing the effective absorbency of the tampons and introducing air at a level to result in toxic shock syndrome.

Chapter 10

Summer 1984 Was Hot, Hot,Hot!

One of the most important and entertaining times in the toxic shock syndrome history was the summer of 1984. Dr. Merlin Bergdoll was organizing a symposium on TSS to be held at the University of Wisconsin, Madison. All or nearly all of the researchers in the field were invited to attend and present their important research. I initially declined to go since I was only given fifteen minutes to speak. Yet for example, Merlin's group had nearly two hours. I refused to participate in such a biased affair. It is my impression, without knowing for sure, that the symposium was to a large extent funded by tampon manufacturers. I say this because when it was found out I was not attending the symposium, I was called by multiple tampon manufacturer representatives to find out why I would not attend. After a short discussion with each, I soon received a phone call from Merlin letting me know I would have more time, an hour if I needed it. I then said I would indeed attend the meeting.

The most important component of the symposium related to the toxin was, or as many investigators called it, "A marker for toxic shock syndrome." There were three orders of business: 1) what was the marker's properties, 2) is it the cause of TSS, and 3) what do we name this maker?

I will start out with the prior observation of my publication in April 1981 *Journal of Infectious Diseases*, where I stated that the toxin pyrogenic exotoxin C (PE C) was the cause of menstrual TSS.[8] Additionally, Merlin Bergdoll's research group published a paper in the non-peer-reviewed journal (at that time) *The Lancet* where he described a protein enterotoxin F in May 1981 and using the biochemical toxin properties I gave him in that unusual phone call to me.[28] I mentioned this in the prior chapter.

I will now present the events of importance that happened at the symposium. Merlin Bergdoll recruited a Canadian investigator Dr. Val Micusan to help him show that the causative toxin had two cysteine amino acids, and thus the toxin should be considered an enterotoxin, which he called enterotoxin F (SEF). The classical staphylococcal enterotoxins have two cysteine amino acids that form a cystine cross-bridge required for vomiting (emetic) enterotoxin activity. The staphylococcal enterotoxins are among the most common causes of food poisoning, characterized by vomiting and diarrhea two to eight hours after eating the toxins. Dr. Micusan presented a complicated story measuring the cysteines, which he found present in very low concentration. The reason for this low concentration will become apparent in a few minutes, but it was the result of contamination. After the Micusan presentation, I pointed out that my laboratory in collaboration with graduate student Barry Kreiswirth and his mentor, Dr. Richard Novick (New York University), showed that there are no cysteines in the toxin, whether you call it C or SEF. Barry made his presentation, providing the complete nucleotide sequence and my laboratory's amino acid sequencing of major, critical parts of the toxin.[55] Indeed, there are no cysteines in the toxin. We knew this then, but our results have been verified by a very large number of studies that have provided the nucleotide sequence of the toxin in hundreds of strains. It is interesting to me that there are no variants of the human toxin, even after all this time. I attribute this to the fact that the toxin is small, 22,000 molecular weight (and not the 20,000 molecular weight number I gave Merlin over the phone). The toxin has the absolute minimum structure needed to have all of its assorted biological activities but notably lacking vomiting activity. As we showed later, it is very difficult to cleave the toxin with proteases, even difficult to cleave the toxin with the small, often-used chemical agent cyanogen bromide, suggesting the toxin is exceptionally tightly folded.[56] I thought there cannot be any variants without losing biological toxicity of the toxin. If it was not toxic, why would the bacteria want to produce it? Its whole role for the bacteria is to cause immune system dysfunction.

The next event of significance was when an investigator with the United States Food and Drug Administration stood up and directly asked: "Merlin, why do you continue to call this toxin an enterotoxin? You and I both know there are no cysteines in the toxin, that it lacks the defining activity, vomiting, and any vomiting activity is associated with a contaminant called staphylococcal enterotoxin A, a toxin that often contaminates the toxin preparations." It turns out that 80 percent of menstrual TSS *Staphylococcus aureus* strains produce both the TSS Toxin and enterotoxin A. They share similar size and similar charge properties, making it very difficult to separate them during purification. It is interesting to me that at a later time, Merlin then switched to purifying TSS Toxin from a *Staphylococcus aureus* strain called FRI 1169. This strain is in the 20 percent that does not produce enterotoxin A.

Thus, we were left with a toxin called PE C or SEF, which had the activities consistent with causing menstrual TSS. However, it was entirely clear to me that the rest of the research community, nearly 250 investigators, were not ready yet to say that this toxin was the cause of menstrual TSS. There then ensued a lot of discussion around this point, and I came to the conclusion that they did not think that Merlin and I could possibly be smart enough to have found the toxin that actually caused menstrual TSS. By this time, I had actually convinced Merlin that we were studying the same toxin; this was difficult, but I got it done. Thus, the rest of the research community continued to call TSS Toxin a marker for menstrual TSS and not necessarily the cause.

Of course, a research group from the TSS task force from CDC wanted to name the toxin, even though they treated me so poorly early on in the TSS epidemic. They wanted to call the toxin Migma Toxin recognizing it was a blend of scarlet fever-like toxin and enterotoxin. They wanted this Migma Toxin to be called a marker instead of cause on menstrual TSS. The problem with Migma Toxin is that just the name alone makes me want to barf. A group from Harvard, of course why would they not be from Harvard, wanted to name the toxin Toxic Shock-Associated Toxin. They also wanted it to be called a marker. Why they should be allowed to name the toxin was beyond me; they were newcomers in the TSS field. The discussion continued for about two hours. To show you just how absurd this discussion became, Dr. John Arbuthnott from Ireland, a long-time researcher in the staphylococcal field, comically and sarcastically suggested TTTWAATA for the name of the marker toxin. This was an acronym for: The Toxin That We Are All Talking About. He clearly was trying to point out the absurdity of this discussion and to get a rise out of the audience. At this point, exceptionally frustrated, I stood up and said: "First of all, if this is not the toxin that causes menstrual TSS and is only a marker, then why does it have all the required toxicity, and why is it the only toxin that all 250 of us are studying?" That had my expected stunning effect on the group, and indeed at this point I got the group to agree that it was the causative toxin.

The next order of business then became naming the toxin. I had originally called the toxin Pyrogenic Exotoxin C (PE C) since pyrogenic toxins were the names of the streptococcal scarlet fever toxins, which share biological toxicity with PE C. I published this in the April 1981 *Journal of Infectious Diseases*. Merlin Bergdoll had named the toxin enterotoxin F (SEF) since he mistakenly thought SEF had emetic activity. His paper was published May 1981 in *The Lancet*. Discussion began with a flurry, and nearly everyone had an opinion. Finally and to his great credit, John Arbuthnott suggested Merlin Bergdoll and I retreat to a private room with a bottle of whiskey and not come out until we had a common name, one with which both of us could agree. To Merlin and me, this was only fitting since we had found the new toxin.

Instead of retreating to a private room, Merlin suggested to the audience that we name the toxin Toxic Shock Toxin (TST). His research technician, for some reason, then literally charged to the front of the room, grabbing the microphone away from Merlin on the way and stated: "I am the person who found this toxin, not Merlin, so I should get to name it." We were all stunned Merlin's research technician would do this to Merlin! The research technician quickly became incomprehensible, so his oration was cut off. He had had a little too much to drink at lunchtime!

The next thing that happened is Dr. Jeffrey Davis, the state epidemiologist for Wisconsin, took the microphone from the research technician and asked for my opinion. I suggested Toxic Shock Syndrome Exotoxin, moving away from PE C which we had used in the above cited manuscript. I pointed out this name would honor Jim Todd who called the disease toxic shock syndrome, and at the same time, I pointed out the protein was an exotoxin (a secreted poison). Merlin and I then acquiesced when Jeff Davis suggested a blending of two names, calling the toxin Toxic Shock Syndrome Toxin (TSST). I agreed right away, and Merlin after some hesitation reluctantly agreed. This then became the name for the toxin on which Merlin and I agreed (TSS Toxin) as I have been using in this book. We published a short paper in the journal *American Society for Microbiology News* and *The Lancet* on the new name.[57]

However, there was one more twist that happened. The rest of the audience wanted a bit more input. What if there was a second TSS Toxin? As I pointed out previously, there never has been, but they wanted input just in case. Thus, the research community adopted the name for this first toxin as TSS Toxin-1. As I said, there never has been a TSS Toxin-2… surprising as this is to me. This then became the name: TSS Toxin-1 (TSST-1). I would no longer use pyrogenic exotoxin C (PE C), and Merlin would retire the name enterotoxin F (SEF).

If I have one regret from the meeting, it is that Merlin and I could have used the glass of whiskey, working so hard to get to this point of agreement. You have no idea! He and I had named the toxin back in 1981, and here we were in the summer of 1984, finally convincing the biomedical community we had the causative toxin of menstrual TSS, and that we had a name for it.

I am never sure why it's so hard for scientists to agree with us, but we were indeed correct. And for the record, this toxin, TSS Toxin, is in fact the cause of 100 percent of menstrual, vaginal-associated staphylococcal TSS. From then on, the rest of the meeting was pretty uneventful. This meeting does portray just how difficult it can be for two strong scientists from public universities, Merlin and me, to convince the world of scientists that we were more than simply dummies, a point I made a long time ago in this book.

Chapter 11

Rocky Mountain West Disease

You now know a lot about menstrual, vaginal staphylococcal toxic shock syndrome. That knowledge will make this chapter a lot easier to understand. In 1987, I was contacted by Dr. Larry Cone (now deceased) of Eisenhower Medical Center, Palm Springs, California, wherein he wanted to publish with me on the possible emergence of a new disease called streptococcal TSS. This was the same disease that I had told the CDC about in August 1980 and for which they blew me off as nonexistent. Of course, I was very much interested in publishing. I performed the toxin testing on the strains of Group A streptococci (*Streptococcus pyogenes*) isolated from two patients with this serious disease. We found the appearance of the original scarlet fever toxin (called scarlet fever toxin A; streptococcal pyrogenic exotoxin A), identified by Drs. George and Gladys Dick way back in 1926. Our collaborative paper was published in the *New England Journal of Medicine* in 1987.[13] In 1989, I was contacted by Dr. Dennis Stevens from Boise, Idaho. He had a larger collection of patients with streptococcal TSS. I again tested the twenty strains from the patients for scarlet fever toxins, and the majority produced scarlet fever toxin A. Along with Dr. Edward Kaplan, University of Minnesota, we published a manuscript describing this disease as the lead article in the *New England Journal of Medicine* in 1989.[14] This paper stands even today as the premier manuscript, cited over one thousand times by other investigators, that describes the expected symptoms, the causative factors, and the therapy. There are few manuscripts as important in any field as this paper is to the health of Americans. I should also remind readers that a manuscript that has been cited forty times is considered high impact in many universities.

There are several things to mention about this disease and particularly, compared to staphylococcal toxic shock syndrome.

Streptococcal TSS is much more severe than menstrual TSS, though it is not any more severe than post-influenza staphylococcal TSS. When originally described, streptococcal TSS was 85 percent fatal, with half of survivors having limbs amputated or major tissue removed. When menstrual TSS was at its peak and only beginning to be recognized, the disease was 30 percent fatal. Post-influenza TSS when we described the disease was 90 percent fatal in children but 100 percent fatal when TSS Toxin was present. Streptococcal TSS appeared first in the United States in the Rocky Mountain West, and this is the basis for the chapter name.

Group A streptococci that cause streptococcal TSS are much more aggressive in causing disease than *Staphylococcus aureus*. What this really means is that the streptococci are more invasive in the body and much more likely to cause serious bloodstream infections, whereas staphylococcal toxic shock syndrome is only occasionally associated with bloodstream infections. I mentioned before that *Staphylococcus aureus* likes to wall itself off from the bloodstream. Additionally, streptococci cause major tissue destruction in what has become known as the flesh-eating disease. Scientists know this as necrotizing fasciitis or necrotizing myositis. The tissue fascia refers to infection of the tissue planes, and myositis means infection of the muscle. When muscle is involved, the cases are nearly always fatal. Necrotizing fasciitis and myositis are quite unusual in staphylococcal toxic shock syndrome, but they occasionally occur. We do not know why Group A streptococci are more invasive than *Staphylococcus aureus*. One thought I have on this is that Group A streptococci do not mind being in the bloodstream. In contrast, *Staphylococcus aureus* seems to want to wall itself off from blood.[58,59] This walling off by *Staphylococcus aureus* may be viewed as a way to allow the bacteria to cause more chronic disease, grow to high numbers, and spread to other people. But remember, Group A streptococcal TSS is incredibly severe and rapidly so. In addition to its high fatality rate, streptococcal TSS patients who survive often have limbs amputated and significant other tissue, for example muscle, removed. I have already mentioned some such cases.

As I said above, streptococcal TSS was first described in the Rocky Mountain West and associated with the scarlet fever toxin A. It appears that the disease moved north from Mexico where it had been hiding out for thirty-five years, waiting for a new, susceptible population to be born. Because of the high mobility of human populations today, the disease became worldwide in no time.

Group A streptococcal strains appear to cycle in the human population in roughly thirty-five-year periods, and this is likely due to the fact that the human immune response to any given strain wanes in thirty-five years. Thus, immunologically naïve humans when exposed to these new strains develop disease. I have mentioned M protein previously in this book. This is a protein on the surface of Group A streptococci that delays white blood cells (the 70 percent PMNs that we have in our bodies) from killing the streptococci. For us to develop the typical "strep throat", the M protein delays these PMNs long enough for us to develop throat damage. There are millions of cases of streptococcal sore throat in the United States each year, usually in children. As I mentioned previously, for some unknown reason, adults seem much less often to develop sore throat due to Group A streptococci.

We know that immunity to Group A streptococci depends on antibodies forming to M protein. Immunity is specific to the M protein of the current disease strain. This means kids can get many Group A streptococcal sore throats. I mentioned in a prior chapter that all Group A streptococcal infections are treated with antibiotics, usually azithromycin today, to prevent delayed sequelae like rheumatic fever. About 5 percent of kids making an immune response to the M protein develop antibodies against M protein that react also with heart tissue and resulting in rheumatic fever. Thus, streptococcal infections are treated with antibiotics to prevent development of antibodies against M protein, where these antibodies, if developed, might react with heart tissue.

It turns out that only certain kinds (as we say M types) of Group A streptococci are associated with certain diseases. When we first described streptococcal TSS, we noticed that cases were nearly always caused by M types 1, 3, and 18; remember there are more than one hundred M types. Interestingly, we also noticed that kids developing strep throat due to these same M types as a rule did not develop streptococcal TSS. I remember one epidemic of "strep throat" in a town in Southeast Minnesota.[60] As many as 35 percent of children in the elementary school had the exact same M type 3 strain in their throats, and they had only "strep throat". However, janitors and other contacts with these infected kids, persons who had breaks in their skin, could get infected with the same M type 3 streptococci and develop streptococcal TSS. There were a total of fifteen cases of streptococcal TSS in this one-town-associated epidemic, and eight died.

At about the same time, I was asked to help with an outbreak of streptococcal TSS in children who had chickenpox. What do children with chickenpox have? Pox lesions that result in breaks in the skin. These cases were associated with M types 1 and 3 streptococci.

I participated in many similar outbreaks with the same observations: these folks were developing streptococcal TSS in association with breaks in the skin. Nearly all of the patients had M type 1, 3, or 18 infections. You could ask why these three M types were so common when there are over one hundred M types. The reason is that these strains make scarlet fever toxin A. Some, 15 percent, of the strains were negative for scarlet fever toxin A, but these 15 percent made another scarlet fever toxin called scarlet fever toxin C. Thus, essentially 100 percent of streptococcal TSS bacteria produce either scarlet fever toxin A or C. This remains true today.

Why don't all Group A streptococcal strains produce scarlet fever toxins A or C, noting by the way that some strains produce both A and C toxins? The reason is that those Group A streptococci that cause streptococcal TSS are infected with a virus that has the toxin gene in its chromosome. These viruses that infect bacteria are called bacteriophages.[41,61] The viruses have very specific receptors on the surface of Group A streptococci that allow only those strains to become infected and in turn, gain the ability to cause streptococcal TSS. The specificity of those viruses explains why M types 1, 3, 18, and occasionally others, streptococci can cause streptococcal TSS. We do not know the receptor on bacteria that the viruses use for infection. Thus, if you think about it, some poor unsuspecting Group A streptococcal strain encounters this nasty virus and becomes infected, and this makes the bacteria cause streptococcal TSS. So... the virus is trying to keep its genes long-term in streptococci by doing this. I should also note that my laboratory is the first laboratory to purify to complete purity these scarlet fever toxins. As I mentioned in an earlier chapter, Lane Johnson, a graduate student, and another graduate student Stephen Goshorn were the first to clone the two scarlet fever toxins so we could understand their function. Through these studies, we showed that the two toxins were highly related to TSS Toxin and the staphylococcal enterotoxins, but immunity to one toxin did not necessarily guarantee immunity to the others.

Streptococcal toxic shock syndrome killed the Muppeteer Jim Henson in 1989. He had a pulmonary infection due to the causative M type 1 streptococcal bacteria. I mentioned that patients with streptococcal TSS most often acquire the bacteria through breaks in the skin. Jim Henson did not. He acquired the streptococci in his lungs. I also mentioned that at that time as many as 85 percent of patients died, and many survivors had limbs amputated and tissue removed. Physicians cannot remove the lungs in patients, so it becomes a real challenge to keep such patients alive.

Believe it or not, all of us know of someone who had streptococcal or staphylococcal TSS. For example, one of my graduate students had recurrent staphylococcal TSS while working in my laboratory. No... she did not acquire the *Staphylococcus aureus* from my laboratory. My father died of staphylococcal TSS following lung infection. While I lived in Minnesota, the brother of one of my neighbors died of staphylococcal TSS. I have also in prior chapters discussed multiple patients with streptococcal TSS whom I helped with disease management.

Let's go back to differences between streptococcal and staphylococcal TSS. There is not a tampon association with streptococcal TSS. As mentioned before, this is the case since Group A streptococci grow and produce their toxins as a function of viral infection but independent of oxygen. Oxygen introduction within tampons explains the association of staphylococcal toxic shock syndrome with tampon use.

The disease definition of streptococcal TSS is basically the same as staphylococcal TSS. However, as mentioned above, streptococcal TSS nearly always has necrotizing fasciitis or myositis as part of the disease, whereas this is rare in staphylococcal TSS. The major difference between the two forms of TSS is that streptococcal TSS is much more aggressive than staphylococcal TSS in progression of symptoms. No one really knows why this difference occurs. Even today, the fatality rate of streptococcal TSS is near 60 percent. Think about it, Ebola is no more lethal than streptococcal TSS, and Ebola infections are not as common as streptococcal TSS. Yet, Ebola infections scare the daylights out of us, but streptococcal TSS does not.

Group A streptococcal TSS only occurs in humans. The reason is that Group A streptococci for some unknown reason can only infect humans. Nearly all cases of streptococcal TSS occur following breaks in the skin, many of which are minor like the above-mentioned chickenpox lesion infections but also like infection of a finger cut as a result of sharpening of ice skates. Remember, I lived for a long time in Minnesota where most kids are born with ice skates on their feet. Think about this, a really minor infection of the skin-cut on a finger can lead to death in two to three days.

I want to mention another neighbor of mine in Minnesota. He developed streptococcal TSS, and he almost died. However, through the heroic actions of his physicians, he survived. About a year later, he developed the disease again, and he almost died again. Upon recovery from the second episode, he called me and asked: "Pat, what can I do to prevent this from happening again?" Here are some things I said to him, and these are generally true with streptococcal TSS. As I do this, I will describe four additional real patients: three children, two of whom died and one of whom survived with three limbs amputated, and one pregnant woman who died and as did her developing fetus. These cases also reflect the very high fatality rate of the disease and how survivors are not left unscathed.

The majority of persons who develop streptococcal TSS acquire the bacteria from other persons, usually kids with pharyngitis. Most of those kids with "strep sore throat" have only that, a sore throat. It is other folks with breaks in the skin who need to worry. Remember, you only acquire this microbe from other people; you cannot blame a pet, and you cannot acquire the microbe from insects or other pests. Humans are the problem source.

It is nearly completely unappreciated that 2 percent of female humans have Group A streptococci vaginally. I teach this to medical students, but I wonder how many retain the information when it is only 2 percent positive. There is also some growing evidence that up to 10 percent of persons with "strep throat" may remain positive for Group A streptococci in the throat long after they are supposedly cured of the microbial infection.

Now, consider: What are the first things that the four patients and my neighbor will experience? They will develop acute, rapid onset of high fever, usually exceeding 102°F, plus they will progressively develop vomiting and diarrhea. These are flu-like symptoms, the same as seen in staphylococcal TSS. The problem with Group A streptococci is that some strains cause disease progression from start to finish in one to three days, whereas others may progress more slowly with start to finish being up to one week. M type 3 and M type 18 strains cause rapid disease progression, whereas M type 1 strains, although also highly fatal, cause a more slowly progressing disease. All of these strains produce scarlet fever toxin A— yes, 100 percent. Let's see how this played out with these four additional patients.

The pregnant woman was a chronic carrier of M type 3 Group A streptococci vaginally, in other words the real baddy. She was perfectly fine until the second trimester of her pregnancy. One day she developed rapid onset of high fever (103.5°F) and vomiting and diarrhea. The next thing she experienced, just like with staphylococcal TSS, is dizziness upon standing. To me, that means she has about twelve hours to live when infected by an M type 3 strain. She recognized that things were not just "the flu" and she immediately went to the local hospital for diagnosis and treatment. She was then admitted because of concern for herself and for the fetus. She was given a bed, and her vital signs were recorded. No disease-causing bacteria were found in her throat, and she did not have any obvious infected breaks in the skin that could account for her symptoms. The hospital staff did not do vaginal cultures, where they would have found Group A streptococci. Also, there is essentially no one left alive or not retired who can routinely test for M type. As I said, this turned out in fact to be an M type 3, found upon autopsy.

I remember this case well because I asked about the blood pressure, temperature, and pulse of the patient. The nurses could not obtain a blood pressure, but they noted the patient appeared to be resting comfortably, even sleeping. Yes, that is true. She was in fact already dead! They could not obtain a blood pressure because she had none, and she appeared to be resting comfortably because what else would dead people do? They noted the patient's temperature was returning to normal, even a bit below expected. Yes, 98°F is a bit below normal. Again, what would be expected of someone who recently died? The most tragic thing, if there could be something worse, is that all of this appeared okay to the nurses since they were able to obtain a pulse of one hundred beats per minute. They then assumed the patient was resting comfortably, as I said. The problem was the fetus's heart was still beating, and what they were measuring was a fetal heartbeat and from a fetus in great distress. The fetus was well on the way to dying in utero, and the fetus did in fact die. Like I said, tragic!

I know of multiple cases just like this in pregnant women. In only one instance did the mother and fetus survive; the disease in that one patient was immediately recognized for what it was, and the fetus was delivered prematurely, with the mother treated with multiple antibiotics and intravenous immunoglobulin, fluid, and electrolytes to keep the blood pressure in the normal range. Remember, these patients can swell up like the Michelin® Tire Man due to blood vessel leak. Thus, it may take a lot of fluid to keep their blood pressure in the normal range. I stated the use of multiple antibiotics. I mention this because streptococcal TSS is usually associated with necrotizing fasciitis and/or myositis. That dead tissue lacks normal blood vessel function, and thus it may be difficult for antibiotics to gain access to the streptococci in the dead tissue and kill them. I mentioned previously that the antibiotic clindamycin has an unusual property of shutting off toxin production even if it is not present in high enough concentration to kill the bacteria. Clindamycin is now standard of care for streptococcal TSS patients. Up to two other antibiotics are also used at the same time as clindamycin. I mentioned intravenous immunoglobulin (antibodies) previously. A now deceased friend of mine Dr. Donald Low, Toronto, Canada showed in a clinical trial that intravenous immunoglobulin can reduce the fatality rate from 85 percent to 30 percent, not perfect but remarkable nonetheless.[62] It should be remembered that persons with this disease do not develop immunity, and although not common, recurrences do happen, just like with menstrual staphylococcal TSS. I know of one case where treating physicians decided to try to administer one-half volume (amount) of intravenous immunoglobulin; this was done because of immunoglobulin cost being $30,000 at that time. The patient started to recover but then fell severely ill again. The patient recovered after the full regimen of immunoglobulin was administered to the patient. I have later shown that the quantity of antibodies to scarlet fever toxin A and C in intravenous immunoglobulin is insufficient unless the entire recommended amount is given to patients.

My neighbor was treated appropriately for his two diseases, just like mentioned above, and then he went on prolonged, preventative therapy with monthly intravenous immunoglobulin to prevent additional recurrences. This worked!

So what about the three children? I want to mention that the disease progression in these kids was the same. They each had a break in the skin that became infected, but the infection site was not inflamed, just like I mentioned occurs with staphylococcal TSS cases. All three kids developed very high fevers, as most kids do, up to 105°F. I will now start with the young girl. Her mother thought: "My child is not behaving normally; she is listless with high fever, so there is something really wrong." She took her daughter in to see the pediatrician daily over the course of a week. Each time, the pediatrician said: "The child has the flu." The mother was instructed to bring the child in if she was not getting better soon. On day seven, all hell broke loose, and the child went into shock. The mother had her daughter transported to a different hospital. The dramatic drop in blood pressure caused clotting to happen in her blood vessels. This could even be seen progressing up her limbs. The child survived but lost three limbs because the blood clotting led to lack of blood, and this meant lack of oxygen in the limbs; the limbs died and became gangrenous. The second hospital in this case did everything correctly. However, the moral of the story is: listen to the mother when she tells you something serious may be going on in her child. Later, the causative bacteria were shown by me to be positive for scarlet fever toxin A, and this was an M type 1 strain.

In the next case, a boy walked into a hospital on his own. He was only seven years old, but he knew something was really wrong with him. He was admitted immediately because he collapsed on the floor. Yes, he was only seven years old. He had a high fever (103.5°F) and low blood pressure... unobtainable. He died a few hours later of M type 3 Group A streptococcal infection.

The third child had a lesion on his left ankle. His disease progressed very rapidly; like I said, that is characteristic of M type 3 and which was the cause of this disease. The child was brought to the Emergency Department of the local hospital with very high fever (107°F), and he appeared extremely toxic. A physician friend of mine saw the patient, and he did everything correct for the therapy. However, tragically as I have said too many times, the child died just a few hours after admission to the hospital. My friend said something really important to me that we should all remember: "Pat, when the patient has an M type 1 infection, that is serious but there is time to get the treatment going. However, when it's an M type 3 disease, the progression is so fast that the physician becomes an absolute wreck, shouting obscenities for not being able to do things fast enough to save the child." Having consulted on over two thousand cases of streptococcal TSS, I agree with him.

There is one other thing to consider here. What do adults do when they don't feel well? If they have flu-like symptoms, they take aspirin or acetaminophen and hope they will feel better in the morning. I have mentioned this before in this book. Streptococcal infections of breaks in the skin will cause pain way out of proportion to the significance of the infection site; they will not show much inflammation. Remember, I mentioned the man who went into a coma for a month. He originally thought he had pulled a muscle, something many of us do periodically (the muscle pull that is). Likewise, we have cuts that may become infected. In all of these cases, the pain that ordinarily would be viewed as way out of proportion to the injury is often masked by the use of aspirin or acetaminophen to reduce pain. I also mentioned that a very high creatinine phosphokinase (CPK) is seen in all TSS patients, whether streptococcal or staphylococcal. This is a sign of muscle damage, it occurs, but we do not have a clue why it occurs. It is a marker of TSS as well as other diseases. Physicians and patients need to be aware of this reduced pain by use of agents like aspirin or acetaminophen.

I want to go back to my neighbor. I mentioned that we all know persons with these diseases. It may seem that I know a lot of sick people. I think of it differently. These folks are taking responsibility for their own bodies, and they and their physicians know that I might be able to help them stay alive. My neighbor again contacted me a few years ago, after I moved to Iowa. He was diagnosed with some form of lymphoma, a tumor of lymphocytes, kinds of white blood cells, and in his case lymphocytes. I think of a line from a song to describe this guy's luck: "Gloom, despair, and agony. Deep dark depression, pain and misery. If it weren't for bad luck, I'd have no luck at all." I heard cast members of the television show *Hee Haw* sing this in a song. I am not sure if they composed it or borrowed it from someone else. Here is where you may listen to it: https://www.youtube.com/watch?v=BkzE23pyME4.

Think about this: Where do lymphomas come from? They occur from multiple mutations in certain white blood cells that lead to one of those aberrant cells becoming malignant and taking over the body. White blood cells must divide lots of times in response to infections over our lifetimes. This is natural. However, with each cell division, there is a rare chance of mutations occurring, only a few of which are needed to lead to tumors. Most of us never develop malignant white blood cells that manifest as lymphoma. However, scarlet fever toxin A, TSS Toxin, and the related family of molecules purposefully dysregulate the immune system by causing massive white blood cell division far out of line of normal. I mentioned that in active menstrual TSS, T lymphocytes that have the correct receptor to bind TSS Toxin divide and become 70 percent of all T lymphocytes in the body. They should only be 10 percent, even in the face of regular infections by microbes. I cannot say that my neighbor developed lymphoma from his two episodes of streptococcal TSS, but it is intriguing. Remember, I said it is never a good idea to be an "interesting patient". However, it is such patients who allow us to learn new things.

Another friend of mine and I published a manuscript where we showed that severe nasal polyps, precancerous growths, are associated with nasal *Staphylococcus aureus* or Group A streptococci that produce the correct pyrogenic toxin superantigens to cause the massive white blood cell division seen in the polyps.[63] Interesting! However, who knows? No one is doing research to find out if there is a connection.

Finally, another friend of mine noticed that some folks with cutaneous T lymphocyte lymphoma, a skin cancer, are infected with the correct *Staphylococcus aureus* to keep this disease going.[64] They produce the correct pyrogenic toxin superantigen, most often TSS Toxin, to keep the lymphoma multiplying. Does TSS Toxin cause the disease, or do people with the disease become infected later with a TSS Toxin-producing *Staphylococcus aureus*? We do not know, but someone should look into this.

I want to address one other issue with streptococcal and staphylococcal TSS related to "interesting" things that merit follow-up, but which are unlikely for follow-up. I am reminded of a twelve-year-old boy, who was seen yearly at a local hospital because of recurrent brain aneurysms that were causing more and more debilitation. I was asked to help since staphylococcal TSS used to be occasionally called Adult Kawasaki Syndrome.[20] Kawasaki syndrome usually occurs in children of Asian descent who are less than four years of age.[22] This syndrome is the greatest cause of acquired heart disease in children; it is associated with significant aneurysms. Aneurysms are weakening of arteries, such that out-pockets occur. These may burst and kill the child. Thus, I was asked to help out to see if this twelve-year-old could have a variant form of TSS (Adult Kawasaki Syndrome). Each time the boy was brought to the hospital, he had a pure culture of TSS Toxin-producing *Staphylococcus aureus* in his throat. Yes, a pure culture. Those of you whom have seen throat cultures for bacteria know that it is highly unusual to find a pure culture. This boy had a disease that resembled Adult Kawasaki Syndrome, wherein aneurysms may be seen. I have also mentioned that TSS patients have many brain dysfunctions for up to one and a half years. Did the TSS Toxin cause this boy's brain aneurysms? As of today, we do not know, but we should. Why not? Read on in the next chapter and you will see why. I have already told you some of the funding problems with staphylococcal TSS, as it relates to diseases of women. I am also reminded of a non-scientist from Texas, where in the summer he says: "It can be hotter than forty acres of burning stumps." At any rate, the man wrote to me, as do lots of folks, because of my time in the news. He said to me in the letter: "Dr. Schlievert, why is it that we know every gene of *E. coli*, we know what every gene does, we know every protein of *E. coli* and what they all do, and we know everything about the metabolism of *E. coli*. Then, why is it that *E. coli* is one of the most dangerous causes of human diseases in the United States and world?" He was absolutely correct in his concerns over *E. coli* and disease. *E. coli* causes 80 percent of urinary tract infections, 1.5 million each year in long-term catheterized patients. Nearly 100 percent of women will have urinary tract infections. At the same time, in the United States nearly one hundred thousand persons will die each year of endotoxin shock (as I mentioned in a prior chapter), and worldwide *E. coli* causes enormous numbers of deaths due to dehydration from diarrheal diseases.

So... how did I answer him? I stated: "You are 100 percent correct to be concerned. I am too. However, you should know that the reason that *E. coli* remains such a bad actor in causing serious diseases is that NIH does not fund grant applications to find out how to manage these diseases. To me, the closer you are to studying human disease, the less likely you are to be funded by NIH to do research."

What Was I Thinking? Toxic Shock Syndrome

I remember submitting a grant to study new diseases and the toxins I thought were causing them. Remember, my colleagues and I have described the causes of twenty-three new infectious diseases. My grant application was turned down with the comment: "Dr. Schlievert's interest in studying new diseases and their causes, although admirable, is not sufficient grounds to have funding from NIH." I also submitted a grant application to the NIH for a novel way to treat *E. coli*-induced endotoxin shock. The grant review panel triaged-out the application, meaning to them the work was not even worth discussing. Keep in mind that my mentor was Dr Dennis Watson at the University of Minnesota. He was THE PERSON in the world who showed how endotoxin works and what part of endotoxin is important. I worked for three years with him, so I have a lot of knowledge of endotoxin. I maintain I am not a complete dummy, even though I have always been a faculty member at a public university. I mentioned this molecule endotoxin made by Gram-negative bacteria in an earlier chapter, where I showed Al Markovetz the structure from *Salmonella*, in too great detail when I was a graduate student; it is part of those Gram-negative bacteria. I don't think it is a coincidence that animals, including humans who can develop TSS whether streptococcal or staphylococcal, are the same ones who are heavily colonized on mucous membranes by endotoxin-containing bacteria. These animals are killed easily by endotoxin. All of the pyrogenic toxin superantigens, including TSS Toxin, the staphylococcal enterotoxins, and the scarlet fever toxins, only cause TSS in the same animals, for example humans and rabbits. Mice cannot develop TSS. I have shown many times that TSS Toxin and these other pyrogenic toxin superantigens amplify the lethal activity of endotoxin by one million-fold.[29] We know that a grain of salt's worth of endotoxin will kill humans. In the presence of TSS Toxin, the amount of endotoxin required to kill a person is one million times less. Have you ever eaten the wrong food and had this "high pressure, nauseating feeling" and followed by explosive diarrhea? That is due to *E. coli* endotoxin leaking into your bloodstream from your large intestine. Come on. We have all had this, so fess up! Now, imagine making that feeling one million times worse. That is TSS!

Finally, leading up to the thoroughly depressing but with a possibly happy ending next chapter, I want you to know that I thought originally of a different title for this book. I thought of the NIH: National Institutes of Health-Less Than Expected. You will see why in the next chapter, the same as I found with menstrual staphylococcal TSS.

There have been many malpractice lawsuits associated with streptococcal toxic shock syndrome since: "Everyone knows Group A streptococci cause the common strep throat, and no one dies of strep throat." What is not recognized is that the Group A streptococci that cause streptococcal toxic shock syndrome have an additional trait that allows them to cause the disease, namely the scarlet fever toxin A.

As noted above, for an unknown reason the majority of cases of streptococcal TSS cases occur in association with the causative bacteria gaining access to the bloodstream through a cut, infection of a chickenpox lesion, or related break in the skin. There are many children with the same bacteria in the throat who develop "strep throat" but not TSS. We do have an appreciation for why M type 3 and 18 strains cause much more rapidly progressing TSS than M type 1 strains, even though both cause serious diseases. M type 3 and 18 strains produce about one hundred times more scarlet fever toxin A per equal unit of time, so the patient is exposed to a lot more toxin early in the disease.

There is significant pain associated with the infection site in streptococcal TSS. In the early stages of infection, many individuals will mask the pain by taking non-steroidal anti-inflammatory agents. This can make diagnosis more difficult. If one looks in the infected tissues, many bacteria can be seen, but cells of the immune system are characteristically absent or present in only low numbers. Thus, the toxin is keeping the immune system at bay.

There is only a small but real chance of recurrence with streptococcal TSS, unlike 40 percent with menstrual toxic shock syndrome. About 20 percent of humans do not make antibodies to the causative toxin. However, women are unique in this regard in that they have menstrual periods once each month. Up to 10 percent of women are colonized vaginally with TSS Toxin-producing *Staphylococcus aureus*. This organism then has the ability to grow vaginally in the presence of menstruation and oxygen in a tampon to result in toxic shock syndrome. In contrast, we consider Group A streptococci to be primary pathogens, and when present in humans, the organisms cause some kind of human disease. In order to prevent development of rheumatic fever, all minor infections, like sore throat, are treated with antibiotics, and the bacteria are eliminated. It would be very unusual to eliminate *Staphylococcus aureus* from human mucosal surfaces.

Larry Cone invited me to Eisenhower Medical Center to give a seminar on streptococcal TSS. At the same time, he invited me to participate in rounds, where I accompanied him on seeing patients with this disease. It was clear that they were very sick and "toxic" looking. However, the most striking thing about the patients was that they looked just like the Michelin® Tire Man in that they were tremendously swelled up. This occurs when fluid leaves the blood vessels, and physicians are trying to keep blood pressure up by giving intravenous fluids to replace fluid lost from the bloodstream. Larry told me that it was not unusual to have to give the patients ten to fifteen liters (quarts) of fluid daily to keep their blood pressure up to normal levels. Remember, if blood pressure drops too much, the organs shut down, and the patient goes into shock and may die.

I worked with Larry on another disease variant of staphylococcal toxic shock syndrome called Recalcitrant Erythematous Desquamating (RED) Syndrome. Recalcitrant means the disease is unrelenting; in the case of RED Syndrome the patients may have seventy-five days of TSS until they die, and 100 percent do die. Erythematous means red skin, like a sunburn or scarlet fever rash. Desquamating means their skin is peeling this entire time. This was a disease that was seen in AIDS patients, and it was always fatal. This disease is not seen much today since drugs are available to manage AIDS. However, it is scientifically interesting to address how this disease could occur. It turns out the major target of the toxins that cause TSS are T lymphocytes. These cells become massively activated by TSS Toxin. Once activated, they are easily infected with the human immunodeficiency virus that causes AIDS. This results in destruction of those T lymphocytes and eliminates the most crucial component of the human immune system. The appearance of new T lymphocytes with their activation by TSS Toxin keeps the process ongoing. This likely accounts for the unrelenting nature of the disease— that is, the reappearance of new T lymphocytes to be activated.

Chapter 12

1989-1993: A Sad State of Affairs?

In the last few years, it has become clear that the NIH grant funding has dropped to the point that many superb investigators are walking away, opting for other career paths or simply retiring. I have said many times that it is very surprising to me that America would spend so much time, so much money, and so much effort to train scientists to such a high level and then torture them for the rest of their lives by making them apply for grants in an impossible system. It is also surprising that we can convince any young person in the United States to pursue a career in biomedical research. Clearly, a part of the problem is that there are insufficient funds available to support the NIH grant system. However, there is a larger, serious problem that is always present but becomes even more prominent at the NIH when funding levels drop to the present levels.

I am convinced that there is a long-standing breakdown in competence and/or ethical standards in many scientists who sit on the NIH grant review panels (called Study Sections) in the NIH branch called the Center for Scientific Review. This breakdown jeopardizes all that we hold as scientifically and medically important. The breakdown often has been actively endorsed by the NIH Center for Scientific Review as well as Journal Editors and other Federal Government organizations. The breakdown results in the lack of self and external scientific recognition that the NIH is supposed to fund research that benefits the health of the American public and not the power and basic science interests of individual investigators or their home universities.

In the next paragraphs, I cite several examples from 1989-1993 that have affected me directly, and I think both adversely impacted the healthcare of the American public and negatively impacted my ability to perform research. These examples demonstrate that many researchers in the scientific community are not interested in human health and further demonstrate a consistent strategy to delay and stop research, that in my case began with identification of TSS Toxin and carrying forward to the present in attempts to develop both a staphylococcal vaccine and novel methods to prevent HIV transmission. This is another small sampling of my experiences, but I have no doubt that many superb, quality scientists have been forced out of research to the detriment of our country's biomedical research.

I will begin by restating a few of my qualifications to make these comments. One way to grade United States researchers is by the impact factor, called H factor, which is a measure of how often others cite the research you have done. An H factor of 40-60 is typical for superb full professors at major universities. H factors above 60 are considered "truly exceptional". My H factor is 98.

My clinical colleagues and I have now described twenty-three novel infectious diseases and have developed important strategies to treat these illnesses. I believe these studies have kept many thousands of Americans and possibly millions alive who otherwise would have died. I have also consulted for no charge on over ten thousand cases of TSS, even though I am not a physician. I believe that my interest in new diseases and their causes, although often given lip service as important by the NIH grant reviewers, is in fact not of interest to them for the NIH funding.

In 2011, I left the University of Minnesota Medical School to become the Head of the Microbiology and Immunology Department at the University of Iowa, Carver College of Medicine. While at Minnesota, I directed and taught 60 percent of the Microbiology and Immunology course for students in training to be physicians. In that capacity, one physician in three who ever trained at the University of Minnesota in its history took Microbiology and Immunology from me. The course was very highly rated.

Now for a presentation on my experience with the NIH with streptococcal TSS about which I think you should know. As I stated in the prior chapter, this is very depressing to think about, but it momentarily did have a happy ending.

At the August 1980 staphylococcal TSS conference in Atlanta, I informed the CDC TSS task force that there was another form of TSS that was caused by *Streptococcus pyogenes* (Group A streptococci) instead of *Staphylococcus aureus*. Because *Streptococcus pyogenes* is an aerotolerant anaerobe, independent of oxygen, I also noted that streptococcal TSS is not associated with tampon use. The CDC TSS task force response was: "There is no such disease." I should also restate two additional pieces of information that affects the discussion of streptococcal TSS. First, the CDC TSS task force approached major journals in the early 1980s, apparently requesting to be the reviewer of all articles on TSS in the interest of "national security". All journals that I know of agreed with the CDC request, except the *Journal of Infectious Diseases*, which of course interfered with the dissemination of science until the *Journal of Infectious Diseases* became the sounding board for science in the TSS field. This also had a major negative impact on my ability to publish studies on TSS.

I think it is telling that I was told by other researchers: "Although you have had major difficulties in publishing studies on TSS due to the CDC, you have made it much easier for us." Second, I had argued strongly with the CDC in 1980 and 1981 that even staphylococcal TSS, not to mention streptococcal TSS, is not necessarily associated with menstruation and tampon use. Indeed, post-menopausal women, children, and males acquire TSS, most often following respiratory viral infection. In 1987, the Minnesota Department of Health and I co-authored a paper in the *Journal of the American Medical Association* describing post-influenza TSS, an illness that was 90 percent fatal in children at that time, and an illness that continues to kill children in the United States each autumn through spring.[6] I estimate that as many as 49,000 children may have died due to this infection since we described it.

In 1987, Dr. Larry Cone's research group at Eisenhower Medical Center and I published an article in the *New England Journal of Medicine* providing the description of streptococcal TSS with/without necrotizing fasciitis.[13] This was followed by the most important and definitive streptococcal TSS study by Drs.

Dennis Stevens and Edward Kaplan and me (and our research groups), published in 1989[14] as the lead article in the *New England Journal of Medicine*. Both of these studies stand today as the premier articles on streptococcal TSS with and without necrotizing fasciitis and myositis, as evidenced by their exceptionally high citation by other authors. Both of these articles again led to intense national publicity, including an episode of the national television show *20/20* with Barbara Walters and Hugh Downs, in which I presented the symptoms, epidemiologic and causative factors, and how to recognize the illness which had become known as "the flesh-eating disease". At that time, streptococcal TSS with necrotizing fasciitis and/or myositis was 85 percent fatal with half of survivors having significant tissue debridement and limb amputations.

As I was studying both staphylococcal and streptococcal TSS, the NIH Study Section grant review panels said: "Dr. Schlievert should separate his studies of the illnesses into different grants since their causation is likely to be different." I took their advice, but this was a mistake. It is for this reason that I remain today non-convinced that rewriting grant applications is helpful to address the non-scientific whims of the NIH Study Sections. At that time, in addition to my ongoing TSS studies, I began studies of three new, but related illnesses caused by streptococci other than *Streptococcus pyogenes*. The consequence of this was that I submitted three grant applications (two renewals and a new application) to the NIH for simultaneous review, all three of which went to the same Study Section (for some unknown reason) grant review panel. These applications studied: 1) staphylococcal TSS, 2) streptococcal TSS, and 3) streptococcal illnesses caused by non-*Streptococcus pyogenes* bacteria. I know today, even though I am not supposed to know, that the same researchers were the principal reviewers on all three applications. The outcome of the review was that all were scored in the 85th percentile, where the 1st percentile is best and 100th percentile is worst. Thus, none of the grants were funded. Furthermore, I was accused of plagiarizing my own grant applications, in that I had used similar writings of methods in all three of the applications. Note again that Study Section had previously asked me to submit these as separate applications, even though most of the methods to be used in the applications were exactly the same. Additionally, I was told in the summary statement (then referred to as pink sheet) of my application for the study of the new illnesses that "the Study Section members looked on *Medline*, and there are no such diseases" and incredibly that "Dr. Schlievert's interest in new diseases and their causes, although admirable, is not sufficient grounds to have funding from NIH".

I have several things to say about the five-year period that followed these reviews. First, I was shocked that none of the applications were funded. This was the second major time, staphylococcal TSS being first, that I had done something absolutely critical to the health of Americans. It was noted by the NIH at that time that streptococcal TSS cost the American healthcare system approximately $1 billion per year. I think I have contributed importantly to bringing those costs down and most importantly, contributed to saving lives. The response to my applications was again to turn down my request for funding. I appealed these decisions to the National Institute of Allergy and Infectious Diseases (NIAID) Council, and the Council asked that the applications immediately be re-reviewed. This was a fair, apparent resolution, but in its wisdom the Center for Scientific Review asked that the same reviewers re-review the applications. It is not surprising that only one was funded, the application related to staphylococcal TSS. The other two remained unfunded. I asked the Scientific Review Administrator for the Study Section why the same reviewers were included, and her response was: "I thought I could force them to be honorable scientists."

At the end of five frustrating years of trying to work within the NIH system for funding the streptococcal TSS research, the National Heart, Lung, and Blood Institute stepped forward, and its lead scientist, Dr. Claude Lenfant (now deceased), said to me in a phone call: "Dr. Schlievert, it does not matter what Study Section says. We will fund your streptococcal grant application." Thankfully, they did. However, I never did receive funding for my studies of the three new diseases that I had by now described in the literature. Instead, other researchers in the United States and other countries were funded to perform the future studies I had initiated. I do not wish to demean the accomplishments of those other researchers, but these were studies I initiated and should have been allowed to complete. I maintain cynically since then that I must have been only lucky to have identified new diseases and their causes, but I am clearly not viewed as smart enough to provide a thorough understanding of how they occur… and thus should not receive funding.

Having provided examples of problems within the Center for Scientific Review, the question becomes: What can be done? The major problem with the center is that for the most part no one holds the Study Section grant reviewers responsible for unethical and incompetent behavior. I think the Center for Scientific Review should be demolished, flattened into nonexistence, and then reconstructed with America's public health in mind. Grant applications should be considered that impact human health, not necessarily directly, but there should be an easily seen impact of the work on human health. Most importantly, Study Section members should be held accountable for their reviews, and if their reviews do not meet ethical and competence standards, those researchers should never be invited back to Study Section and should never again be allowed to participate in the NIH grant application system.

It is stated that the NIH has difficulty attracting high-quality reviewers today, and that is what explains the poor reviews that many researchers receive. The way to deal with this issue is to make incentives for strong, ethical researchers to review grants. This should be done through incentivizing a small group of perhaps ten reviewers for the duration of their doing grant reviews for individual Study Sections. Hold these researchers responsible for doing a good job. In all other aspects of American lives, we are asked to do assessments of the quality of our work, and we are expected to perform well. The same should be done of the Center for Scientific Review.

Chapter 13

2012-2014

This is the next to the last chapter, where I will take you through some of my additional recent shocking experiences in dealing with the NIH grant-funding system. Again in 2012, I was required to renew my grant to study streptococcal TSS. As I could expect, the Study Section grant review panel recommended that my grant application for continued funding be turned down. They had three major negative comments.

First, it was stated: "Dr. Schlievert must be heavily involved with administrative work because he has not been as productive as usual." Indeed, I had just become the chair of the Microbiology and Immunology Department at the University of Iowa. However, lack of productivity? Let's see: Most researchers publish at most two manuscripts per year related to any given grant. Grants are most often funded for five years, but a renewal must be submitted at the four-year-and-three-month time point to ensure continued funding, funding without disruption of ongoing research and to maintain research technician salaries. If you do not receive continued funding, you will need to lay off employees and most importantly stop the research. So, the average researcher would publish about nine manuscripts in that four-year-and-three-month period of funding. I had published forty-two manuscripts, many of which have already become high impact. So, productivity was not really a problem. The comment from the Study Section was in fact nonsense.

The second comment was: "Dr. Schlievert is not keeping up with the epidemiology of *Staphylococcus aureus* infections. He proposes to continue his studies of multiple strains, when we know for certain that USA300 MRSA strains are the most important to be studying. Furthermore, USA200 strains that produce TSS Toxin are becoming unimportant." In fact, I have been keeping up on epidemiology. As I have stated in prior chapters, strains of *Staphylococcus aureus* come and go in roughly ten-year intervals, so it is important to study multiple strains. I had already published many manuscripts where I studied the common strains with CDC designation, including USA100, USA200, USA300, and USA400. This culminated with a publication in 2014 where my laboratory successfully vaccinated rabbits against *Staphylococcus aureus* pneumonia.[65] There are seventy thousand human cases of staphylococcal pneumonia each year, and nearly 60 percent will die from this infection. That is forty-two thousand deaths. I thought at the time and I think today that we can develop a staphylococcal vaccine by targeting the pyrogenic toxin superantigens, including TSS Toxin and enterotoxins B and C. This is what was done in the large publication in 2014 *Journal of Infectious Diseases.*

It has been well known since 1980 that I think USA200 strains of *Staphylococcus aureus* are important. These are the strains that produce TSS Toxin, and they cause 100 percent of menstrual, vaginal TSS and 50 percent of non-menstrual, staphylococcal TSS. As you by now know, I think pyrogenic toxin superantigens are the toxins that kill humans, and this is why persons die of *Staphylococcus aureus*. I have shown this in multiple publications with use of rabbits as the animal model. This thought bothers many scientists, because if pyrogenic toxin superantigens are so important in human disease, then it would mean that those investigators should be required to change their area of emphasis to study the toxins. This, they clearly do not want to do.

I have also already mentioned the many failed human vaccine trials against *Staphylococcus aureus*. Why was the last one even done, which resulted in five times as many vaccinated persons dying, compared to non-vaccinated persons? I had already published why this vaccine trial would fail. Yet, some researchers as I have mentioned have "extra connections", and they do not have to listen to the rest of us, regardless of the important scientific data we have.

There was one other mitigating factor that allowed the NIH grant review panel to make the statement to the effect that I was not keeping up with the epidemiology of the day. A collaborative group of researchers had published a paper in the *Proceedings of the National Academy of Sciences*. Originally, I was supposed to be included as a co-author on the manuscript. We had made this decision at an important Gordon Research Conference. I am not sure why the paper was published as it was, but I was not included as an author, and I would never have approved its submission. I had sent 100 USA200 *Staphylococcus aureus* strains to the collective group of investigators. Remember, these are the strains that cause TSS due to production of TSS Toxin. I had sent all of the strains as obtained from otherwise healthy persons who then developed TSS, and wherein 30 percent had died of their disease. Most importantly, none of these strains came from persons who had been originally in hospitals with immune compromised states, for example with treatment for cancer. None had!

The essence of the *PNAS* manuscript was to show that newly emergent skin strains of *Staphylococcus aureus* were more virulent than the USA200 TSS Toxin-positive strains. The newly emergent strains were the USA300 strains that cause large skin abscesses and boils, and occasionally they cause fatal pneumonia. The USA200 strains included those provided by me.

With this as background, the authors were thus comparing apples and oranges. They did not recognize that it makes no sense to compare the virulence of skin strains versus mucous membrane strains of *Staphylococcus aureus*. I have already told you that USA200 strains cause menstrual TSS due to TSS Toxin. I have also told you that these strains killed 30 percent of infected persons. These strains also produce very little alpha toxin, a poison required for *Staphylococcus aureus* USA300 strains to cause skin infections. Thus, one cannot compare USA300 skin strains to USA200 mucous membrane strains for ability to cause the same diseases.

Next, these investigators compared the USA300 and USA200 strains in a mouse model of pneumonia, and guess what? The USA300 strains had better ability to cause disease. This should be no surprise to anyone, since I had already published many times that TSS Toxin and related pyrogenic toxin superantigens are NOT toxic to mice.[12] Thus, mice do not develop TSS. Of course, this can be ignored if the present investigators choose to ignore the prior data, which they did.

I had already told them at our meeting at the Gordon Research Conference that researchers cannot test USA200 strains in mice, since mice do not develop TSS. In fact, I have found that the production of TSS Toxin by USA200 strains of *Staphylococcus aureus* renders mice less susceptible to infection, the opposite of what is seen in humans, and rabbits as the model.

The worst thing the authors of the paper did, however, was state that USA200 strains are found only in immune compromised patients in hospitals. I have already told you that none of the one hundred strains I sent the authors for use in studies came from immune compromised patients in hospitals. How could they have stated this? I certainly don't know!

Many journals allow other researchers to challenge the findings of published manuscripts by writing a letter to the editor pointing out what is wrong with the manuscript. Many researchers ask me why I did not write such a letter if I had information that said the findings in the paper were wrong. In fact, I DID submit a letter to the editor, but it was not published, for a reason unknown to me. It is provided in its entirety in the following paragraphs, though I have removed the authors' names. I have also omitted my supporting references, but if you want those references, I am happy to provide them.

The "First Author et al." study contains inaccuracies. *Staphylococcus aureus* strains cycle, often in hospitals, in ten-year intervals. However, there is no required high to low-virulence adaptation with cycling. This is contrary to the study that indicates epidemic 80/81 and common USA200 strains, while sharing ancestry, diverged with 80/81 retaining high virulence while USA200 strains attenuated through Agr (*agr*C) and α-toxin gene mutations.

USA200 (known as 29/52) and 80/81 strains were simultaneously present in humans during the 1950s 80/81 epidemic. USA200 strains were already mucosal-adapted, being α-toxin^{low+}, whereas 80/81 strains were skin-adapted, being α-toxin^{high+}. This was not USA200 virulence reduction compared to 80/81, but rather preexistent organism adaptation to different niches. For one hundred years α-toxin has been known to be required for *S. aureus* skin survival; mucosal isolates produce one hundred times less α-toxin.

The authors suggest that USA200 strains are attenuated, causing illnesses in compromised persons. USA200 strains are known to cause serious illnesses in previously healthy persons. The plague of Athens (430-429 BC) may represent post-influenza toxic shock syndrome (TSS) caused by USA200, as recognized in 1987 when several children succumbed. There was also significant emergence of USA200 in 1970 that led not to attenuation but instead to increased virulence. The superantigen TSST-1 was produced by <10 percent of USA200 prior to 1970, but emerged to >85 percent by 1975 with consequent TSS epidemic.

The "First Author et al." suggest mutation of *agrC* in USA200 contributes to reduced virulence. TSST-1 is tightly regulated by *agr*, with twenty-fold reductions in TSST-1 in *agr-* versus *agr+* strains. However, TSST-1 production by *agrC* mutant USA200 is high; women may have one hundred μg on tampons, and in vitro biofilms may contain twenty mg/ml (<1 μg/human can be lethal).

In 1980, USA200 colonized 5 percent of humans. Today, 25 percent are colonized on mucosal surfaces. Considering 40 percent have mucosal *S. aureus*, 60 percent of colonized humans have TSST-1+ strains. Nearly 80 percent of hospital infections result from nasal *S. aureus*, indicating USA200 strains are the most common infection strains. These strains do not infect intact skin due to α-toxin[low+], but cause serious post-surgical infections where organisms gain access to skin breaks. The organisms also cause pneumonia TSS and are common causes of persistent bacteremia in endocarditis. I sent nearly 100 TSST-1+ USA200 to the authors from patients with serious/fatal TSS. The strains are included in their studies.

I question the use of mouse testing to assess virulence. We can agree without experimentation that 80/81 and USA200 strains will exhibit virulence differences. Mice can be killed by α-toxin from skin 80/81 strains but are resistant to TSST-1 produced by USA200 strains.

The "First Author et al." also study α-toxin in serious illnesses caused by currently emerging skin strains that accordingly are α-toxin[high+]. Studies suggest that vaccination against these strains in mice is achieved by immunization against α-toxin. In order for such a vaccine to be of general use, USA200 strains must become unimportant.

The above paragraphs were it, my letter to the editor of the *Proceedings of the National Academy of Sciences*.

I believe now that this *Proceedings of the National Academy of Sciences* manuscript is the ONE that the reviewers on the NIH grant review panel were referring to when they said: "Dr. Schlievert is not keeping up." The reviewers' names are supposed to be kept confidential, but leaks happen in the Federal Government, and I know who the first two major reviewers were. This is what I would expect from them.

I mentioned three criticisms. The third one is completely absurd, as if the above ones were not absurd enough. The reviewers criticized MY use of mice in research. Anyone, even you who have read the book up to this point, will know that I DO NOT use mice in research. Mice are simply not susceptible to TSS, so why would I use an irrelevant model?

I did appeal the grant review panel decision not to fund my continued research. I appealed to the appropriate component of the NIH, the National Institute of Allergy and Infectious Diseases Council. The council said the reviews were perfectly fine. I resubmitted the grant application twice more, responding to the reviewer comments. The grant has never been renewed, and I have stopped doing research in this area. What has that meant to you as Americans?

What I now see happening is that the fatality rate for both staphylococcal and streptococcal TSS is increasing. There is less and less recognition of these important diseases, to a large extent because I am no longer keeping them in the public eye. This aspect is very discouraging to me, as I have devoted my entire research career doing things to help the American public. This is now ended! Sorry! If the NIH no longer cares about your health, why or how should I care?

I will have one more chapter that addresses things we have shown. I will also comment more on what I think needs to be done for the future of *Staphylococcus aureus* and Group A streptococcal research. I will leave it up to you to decide if I am correct.

Chapter 14

Where Do We Go Now?

Good question! I wish I knew. I will tell you what I have recently been up to, and then tell you what I think should happen next, and perhaps you should tell me what's next since the Federal Government and science are clearly not listening to me.

As I have said, my clinical colleagues and I have described a total of twenty-three new diseases, what we thought and now know causes them, and how we can manage them. We have more recently done a lot of studies relative to diabetes mellitus type II and infective endocarditis. Finally, I have some wonderful collaborators on other new diseases associated with TSS Toxin-producing *Staphylococcus aureus*.

I want to return briefly to the staphylococcal alpha toxin story with Sir Macfarlane Burnet in Bundaberg, Australia. I have already told you that Dr. Burnet suggested that this alpha toxin killed twelve of twenty-four children exposed to diphtheria and who were given staphylococcal-contaminated horse-antibodies raised against diphtheria toxin. I also told you that an undergraduate and graduate student in my laboratory showed the Bundaberg *Staphylococcus aureus* strain killed the children, not due to alpha toxin but instead due to TSS Toxin. What I now want to tell you is more of the sordid in-depth story.

Since 1928, staphylococcal alpha toxin has been far and away the MOST heavily studied toxin of *Staphylococcus aureus*. There have been thousands of manuscripts published suggesting its great importance in human diseases. Indeed, this toxin was the center of the solar system. It was even the center of the Milky Way galaxy. Possibly, it was the center of the universe.

However, the Bundaberg *Staphylococcus aureus* do not even produce alpha toxin. Dr. Burnet did a bait-and-switch on us that led to that thinking. He was completely unable to show that the Bundaberg *Staphylococcus aureus* produced alpha toxin, so he tested other staphylococcal strains. He found these other strains to produce this new toxin which he called alpha toxin. Then, he said alpha toxin must be causing the deaths of the children. As you know by now, those alpha toxin-producing *Staphylococcus aureus* strains were not producing TSS Toxin. Since Dr. Burnet was such an important scientist, the father of modern immunology after all, everyone believed him... that is that alpha toxin caused the children's deaths. This thinking persisted up until a few years ago when my students studied the Bundaberg strain. Imagine how many times I have had to put up with researchers telling me that alpha toxin is so important, and TSS Toxin is so unimportant? Too many is the number. My experience is that most of the grant review panel scientists do not have the foresight to be reviewing grants, much less reviewing manuscripts.

When the undergraduate, graduate student, and I published our manuscript, it was not in one of the premier journals such as the *Nature* group.[27] Indeed, there are many alpha toxin manuscripts published in the *Nature* group, almost certainly because the "correct, pretty" people were studying that toxin and knew with great certainty that it was important. Our manuscript was published in a European journal called *Microbiology*, published there since we knew the Europeans were honest scientists and would give it a fair review. Our thinking also was that the United States research community was too heavily invested in alpha toxin to have it become unimportant... which it mostly is. These days when I speak about my two students, I tell everyone that they put the sun back in the center of the solar system, a black hole back in the center of our galaxy, and TSS Toxin back in the center of the universe where it belonged all along. Think about this: What would be different today if Sir Macfarlane Burnet had described TSS Toxin back in 1928? A lot of young women, mothers and daughters, would not have died.

Many of you will find it hard to believe, but scientists like Isaac Newton and Charles Darwin were arrogant, political jerks, not at all honorable scientists. Elsewhere in this book, I stated that scientists are not so different from all humans, many are even much worse because of their self-elevated sense of importance. I honestly believe this to be your detriment.

There are, however, many honorable scientists, including some who I have named in the book: my friends Mike Osterholm, Jeff Parsonnet, Roger Stone, Donald Leung, Gary Dunny, Pat Cleary, Robert (Bob) Coates, Malak Kotb, Marnie Peterson, and Catherine Davis. I appreciate them all! I do not require lots of friends. I just need some good ones, and these are good ones. I just wish Gary Dunny and Bob Coates had each not made me run eighteen thousand miles over eighteen years; that's thirty-six thousand miles, guys.

I have already discussed in detail staphylococcal and streptococcal TSS, and I have briefly mentioned to you that non-Group A streptococci also occasionally cause streptococcal TSS. I would now like to address extreme pyrexia syndrome for a few minutes.

A very good friend of mine, an infectious diseases physician originally from South Dakota and not "South Athens Greece" by the name of Dr. Aris Assimacopoulos called me one day about patients he had seen. These patients were infected with *Staphylococcus aureus* that produced what appeared to be a remnant of TSS Toxin. These patients presented to the hospital with fevers of rapid onset and going above 108°F. The fevers remained high, despite heroic efforts to bring the fevers down, including with cold fluids and ice baths. Humans cannot stand fevers this high, and the patients died rapidly. Several other similar cases have been reported to me, and as above, 100 percent have died rapidly.

This is one of only a few diseases that I have been associated with where the fatality rate remains the same as when identified... at 100 percent.[17] In all other instances, the fatality rate has dropped. This one remains 100 percent fatal as I said. At this time, I know only that *Staphylococcus aureus* causes the disease. I do not know the role if any of the TSS Toxin is remnant. I do not know why fever rises so fast and so high. I know how fever occurs, as I told you early on in this book. However, what triggers such a fast and high fever is beyond my understanding at this time. I would like to know if it is a staphylococcal factor that is causing such a high fever, or alternatively if it is a group of humans who are genetically predisposed to high fever. At this point, I wish someone could figure this out. I no longer have funding to do so.

Another infectious diseases physician friend of mine Dr. Gary Kravitz and I described a new disease caused by *Staphylococcus aureus*, a disease called staphylococcal purpura fulminans.[66] This is a rapidly-progressing (fulminans), toxin-induced disease that has high fever, significant drop in blood pressure, and blood leaving the vessels in large amounts, causing purple legs, arms, and trunk (purpura). When we described this disease, it was 75 percent fatal and mostly caused by MRSA. Like extreme pyrexia syndrome, this is a terrible disease and requires superb physicians to recognize what is going on with the patients. With recognition of the disease, and optimal physician care, the fatality rate has dropped to 25 percent. This is a great start.

At this time, we know pyrogenic toxin superantigens kill the patients, but we do not know why they develop the purpura, and we do not know why the purpura occur so fast. We know that two other bacteria also cause this. Yes, you guessed correctly Group A streptococci are one of them. These bacteria obviously also produce pyrogenic toxin superantigens. The other bacteria that are common causes of purpura fulminans are *Neisseria meningitidis*. This has been known for a long time. We even know how that disease occurs. The *Neisseria meningitidis* are Gram-negative bacteria so they have endotoxin. The bacteria gain access to the bloodstream and very rapidly cause overwhelming endotoxin shock. One aspect of endotoxin shock is something called disseminated (meaning spread throughout the body) intravascular (meaning within the blood vessels) coagulation (meaning clotting), or as it is often called DIC. DIC blocks blood flow to organs and tissues, which blocks oxygen getting to the organs and tissues. The blood vessels die due to lack of oxygen, and blood massively leaks into the adjacent tissue, leading to purpura. I mentioned to you that animals with dominant Gram-negative normal microbiome are the ones who develop staphylococcal and streptococcal TSS. Thus, maybe staphylococcal purpura fulminans happens because of the impressive synergy between TSS Toxin and intestine-derived endotoxin. If that is true, and I think it is, then why do not all TSS patients develop purpura fulminans? We simply do not know. I likewise am not funded to find out what exactly is going on so we can develop better treatments and get the fatality rate to zero.

I have spent a significant amount of my recent time looking at the role of pyrogenic toxin superantigens in known staphylococcal and streptococcal diseases. I will summarize most of this with one sentence: These toxins are required for *Staphylococcus aureus* and Group A streptococci to cause ANY disease. I will discuss staphylococcal infective endocarditis for a few paragraphs.

Infective endocarditis is an infection of the heart, often the heart valves, leading to the valves not working properly. There are one hundred thousand cases of infective endocarditis in the United States each year. Nearly forty thousand of those cases are caused by *Staphylococcus aureus*. The staphylococcal cases are typically highly severe and rapidly progressing. The time from infection to death may be as short as a few days. Patients with this serious infection also have other trouble. They develop strokes due to pieces of the destructed heart valves, tissues, and bacteria breaking off and getting stuck in the brain. This results in clots that in turn destroy the brain blood vessels and leads to hemorrhages and resultant strokes. Other things that commonly happen are pulmonary (lung) clots and metastatic (spread) staphylococcal infection throughout the body. No wonder the fatality rate is greater than 50 percent for this disease. We have shown in the rabbit model that the pyrogenic toxin superantigens are critical for causing this disease. In what way, do we not know? A former postdoctoral associate of mine Dr. Wilmara Salgado-Pabón is pursuing this.

It turns out that non-Group A streptococci and enterococci, bacteria related to Group A streptococci, cause the remaining sixty thousand cases of infective endocarditis each year. We have studied these more slowly progressing, yet highly fatal diseases. We know that pyrogenic toxin superantigen-like molecules are important. How so? We simply do not know.

We have also examined the possible role of pyrogenic toxin superantigens like TSS Toxin and enterotoxins B and C in diabetes mellitus type II. We have been able to produce diabetes mellitus type II in our rabbit model.[26] There are about thirty million people in the United States with diabetes mellitus type II. In our studies, we have shown that people with this form of diabetes have about ten trillion *Staphylococcus aureus* on their skin. Think about it this way. Make a square by putting your forefinger and thumb together. This is about the size of a quarter stick of margarine. That is the same as about ten trillion *Staphylococcus aureus*. Something that is unusual is that those bacteria produce one of TSS Toxin, enterotoxin B, or enterotoxin C. We could measure the amounts of these toxins on the skin of people, which we did. Then, we administered that amount of toxins chronically to rabbits. Guess what? They developed the required symptoms of diabetes mellitus type II: failure to remove sugar from the blood, insulin-resistance, and fatty liver. We would like to know two things: 1) how does this happen, and 2) why do people with diabetes type II select for pyrogenic toxin superantigen-producing *Staphylococcus aureus*? If we knew the answer to these questions, we might be able to convince the world that these findings are cause and effect and not simply coincidence. If you remember, I went through the same experience with showing TSS Toxin is in fact the cause of TSS. I do have some funding to pursue this research.

My friend Dr. Donald Leung, National Jewish Health, and I have worked together for a long time, both studying the cause of atopic dermatitis and Kawasaki Syndrome. Atopic dermatitis is essentially a skin disease that is a severe form of eczema, which can significantly alter the lives of affected persons. There are some forms such as eczema herpeticum that can be life threatening. It is clear to me that staphylococci cause this atopic dermatitis, but the question is how. That is what we are funded to examine.

I have mentioned that staphylococcal TSS occasionally used to be called Adult Kawasaki Syndrome, when no one knew what TSS was. So, what then causes Kawasaki Syndrome? Donald Leung and I have been examining the possible role of *Staphylococcus aureus*.

It makes sense to consider *Staphylococcus aureus* for many reasons. Here is what we know so far. Adult Kawasaki Syndrome and Kawasaki Syndrome have overlapping symptoms, and that is why they were so named. Kawasaki Syndrome generally occurs in children less than four years of age, and Adult Kawasaki Syndrome occurs in older individuals and is TSS.

I gave a symposium address at an Infectious Diseases Society of America (not the one on TSS), where I was supposed to explain the difference between Kawasaki Syndrome and TSS. When I finished with my address, a researcher from Chicago who studies Kawasaki Syndrome said to me: "Pat, you did a good job explaining TSS versus Kawasaki Syndrome, but I would like to emphasize that there are two differences between Kawasaki Syndrome and TSS. Kawasaki Syndrome patients develop middle-sized blood-vessel aneurysms, whereas TSS patients do not. TSS patients develop hypotension and shock, whereas Kawasaki Syndrome patients do not."

However, the next questioner emphasized: "I have just seen three adult women with TSS, and all three had coronary artery aneurysms, so you cannot use development of aneurysms to separate the diseases." I would also like to say that Dr. Chet Whitley and I tried to publish a manuscript on infant TSS. We were never allowed to do this because some of the defining clinical features of TSS were missing. Thus, if hypotension is the missing symptom, then the infants have what looks exactly like Kawasaki Syndrome.

Some of my clinical friends think the rash of TSS and Kawasaki Syndrome are different. Others say that you cannot tell the difference. Let me remind you of the boy who was seen yearly and who developed brain aneurysms in association with throat infections by TSS Toxin-producing *Staphylococcus aureus*. I will also give you a few other pieces of data that Donald Leung and I have collected. First, TSS patients respond well when intravenous immunoglobulin is added as part of the therapy. I have mentioned this therapy multiple times previously. Kawasaki Syndrome treatment always includes intravenous immunoglobulin as well.

I was called by a surgeon in Kansas several years ago. His daughter was infected with *Staphylococcus aureus*, but she was diagnosed with Kawasaki Syndrome. The diagnosis of Kawasaki Syndrome includes the lack of response after a week of antibiotics to treat bacterial infections. As I have mentioned in prior chapters, many women develop recurrences of TSS despite antibiotic therapy. It is very difficult if not impossible to "cure" someone of *Staphylococcus aureus*. We do not know all the reasons why, but I can think of at least three: 1) the microbe can hide out in body sites where antibiotics cannot penetrate; 2) the microbe may be an MRSA (I know of multiple menstrual TSS patients with incomplete treatment for failure to recognize that some menstrual TSS microbes are MRSA); and 3) the person may be cured of *Staphylococcus aureus* and then re-infected (40 percent of all humans are infected with this microbe). Thus, it is not surprising that the surgeon's daughter's Kawasaki Syndrome did not respond to antibiotic therapy. The surgeon said to me: "Pat, if you can show that the Kawasaki Syndrome is being caused by TSS Toxin *Staphylococcus aureus*, then I can tell this to her treating physicians, gain much more aggressive antibiotic therapy for TSS, instead of just giving intravenous immunoglobulin for Kawasaki Syndrome." He sent me the *Staphylococcus aureus* by Federal Express, and the next day (the day the sample arrived) I told him the microbes produced TSS

Toxin. Remember, I mentioned previously that I recommend three antibiotics at a time for TSS cases: vancomycin in case of MRSA, clindamycin since this antibiotic shuts off TSS Toxin production, and rifampin since it penetrates better into hidden sites. The surgeon's daughter recovered.

I participated in two blinded studies related to the cause of Kawasaki Syndrome. I received twenty coded samples of blood from Kawasaki Syndrome provided to me by Dr. Kawasaki, the physician researcher after whom the disease was named. I assayed the samples to see if the children who had Kawasaki Syndrome and then recovered tested positive or negative for antibodies to TSS Toxin. When the code was broken, none of ten of the children with Kawasaki Syndrome active disease was positive for antibodies, meaning they were susceptible to TSS Toxin. Upon recovery from the disease, five of ten of the children developed antibodies to TSS Toxin. This means that at least these five had been recently exposed to TSS Toxin. One-half did not develop antibodies upon recovery. Remember that I told you, by twelve years of age, the decision has been made as to whether your body can make antibodies to TSS Toxin. Thus, some of these children would be expected to be able to produce antibodies to the toxin upon recovery, but 20 percent would not produce antibodies.

I also participated in another, much larger study, in which cultures were taken from multiple body sites from children with Kawasaki Syndrome and compared to children without Kawasaki Syndrome. The cultures were sent both to the regular CLIA-certified diagnostic laboratories and to me; I did all the testing of samples sent to me by myself. The patient groups came from multiple geographic sites in the United States. When the code was broken there were two things that stood out to me. First, the CLIA-certified laboratories DID NOT find *Staphylococcus aureus* in the children. How could this have been, when 40 percent of children typically are infected with *Staphylococcus aureus*? I found *Staphylococcus aureus* present in all except one Kawasaki Syndrome child, the one exception being positive for Group A streptococci. This is important! Why did the diagnostic laboratories NOT find *Staphylococcus aureus*? I know the answer. I kept my samples for seven days, but the diagnostic laboratories did not retain theirs. It turns out *Staphylococcus aureus* that when cultured in the laboratory on what we call blood agar plates (good growth media for many bacteria), other bacteria can suppress the growth of *Staphylococcus aureus*. Only later on, perhaps four to five days, can *Staphylococcus aureus* appear.

I have also told you that being an "interesting patient" is never a good idea. A friend of a friend of mine had a recurrent disease that resembled TSS, one of these "interesting patients". His disease appeared each summer, which often happens with both staphylococcal and streptococcal TSS for some unknown reason. I was asked to help with this patient. Did he have a variant form of TSS? Cultures were taken, and I grew the cultures on typical blood agar plates (by the way, this is sheep blood not human blood). I saw nothing that resembled *Staphylococcus aureus* until day four. I have this purely-isolated *Staphylococcus aureus* in my laboratory, and it always grows slowly.

While getting my PhD in Microbiology and Immunology, I took a diagnostic microbiology course that lasted five months. I worked all day long at each station in the laboratory, testing samples from all over Iowa for various bacteria. One thing I quickly learned was that most diagnostic laboratories assume *Staphylococcus aureus* will form visible colonies in less than twenty-four hours, so less than one day. This is clearly to me not true from what I saw in the Kawasaki Syndrome studies.

I would also like to comment on identification of Group A streptococci, since one of the Kawasaki Syndrome children was positive for this microbe. I am reminded of an outbreak of "sore throat" in the college student population at a major university. No Group A streptococci were found. This made no sense to me, since I found Group A streptococci in the throats of 100 percent of the students. I later found out that the diagnostic laboratory was not set up properly to find Group A streptococci. When they followed my advice and changed procedures, they too then always found Group A streptococci. This is important as I hope you recognize, since all persons with Group A streptococci must be treated with antibiotics to prevent them from developing the autoimmune disease rheumatic fever. And I am the one not-CLIA certified!

I found one other thing in the large blinded study. I found that the majority of *Staphylococcus aureus* from the Kawasaki Syndrome children produced TSS Toxin, whereas the *Staphylococcus aureus* from non-Kawasaki Syndrome children did not produce the toxin.

Thus, from this study and combined with all other data, I felt then and still do now that many cases of childhood Kawasaki Syndrome are caused by TSS Toxin-producing *Staphylococcus aureus*. What do I need to do yet to prove this? I need to develop an animal model which duplicates production of aneurysms by TSS Toxin.

Then and only then, I think I could win the day. However, the NIH does not appear interested in this research since many (90 percent), but not all, Kawasaki Syndrome patients respond well to intravenous immunoglobulin.

One final research project that I have small funding for is to find out why oxygen is absolutely required for TSS Toxin production. If we can understand this, it is possible we can find things to add to tampons to prevent TSS Toxin production.

I would now like to switch to the final and most important aspect of this book. What is important to remember, and what do we do next?

First and foremost, all persons in the world should know what the symptoms of TSS and its possible variants might be. It is not the flu if you have a fever of greater than 102°F, vomiting and diarrhea, and dizziness upon standing. This is a sign of impending doom, and you should immediately get to a hospital before you pass out. Be sure to mention to physicians that you think you may have TSS, either staphylococcal or streptococcal. Keep in mind that there are many variants of TSS. Children do not develop acute-onset rheumatoid arthritis for no reason. *Staphylococcus aureus* TSS Toxin is likely causing this. You will need to take care of yourself and not just say: "Doctor, make me well." There are really good physicians out there, but there are many who are not so good. The best way to tell is to have an idea of what is wrong with you and why you are coming in. You can judge their response.

When I first publicized staphylococcal TSS in 1980, it was only fortunate that I was a faculty member in California. The news media pay a lot of attention to news from the coasts but not so much for the Midwest... even though we have important things to say. With the media attention, I was able to tell America and then the world about TSS. For example, we now have uniform labeling of tampons all over the world according to absorbency. There is no more Tampax® Super being the second lowest absorbency tampon on the market and Playtex® Regular being higher absorbency than Tampax® Super. All absorbencies are standardized, regardless of country. Additionally, the very high absorbency tampons have been removed from the market. Women are advised that if they want to reduce their risk of menstrual TSS not to use tampons. However, if they choose to use tampons, they should use the lowest absorbency to control menstrual flow, and they should change the tampons every four to eight hours.

From the time after the mid-1990s that news media attention has waned, TSS has not gone away. However, many folks including physicians think it has because it is not in the news as much. I was able to keep TSS in the minds of America for a long time by issuing press releases on new findings. I am no longer funded in the area of TSS research. I note that an NIH program officer in the National Institute of Allergy and Infectious Diseases recently said to me: "Pat, what have you done for us recently? That is why you cannot get your grant funded." I am not sure what he meant, but it was a dumb statement! I took his comment to mean, that since I am interested in human diseases, their causes and how the diseases happen, and how we can keep people alive, this does not merit funding. I should note that it is NOT his job to decide funding; it is the responsibility of the Center for Scientific Review at the NIH.

For a long time, I used to send in op-ed letters to major newspapers to let them know that TSS following influenza is deadly. These letters are no longer published, so I have stopped. However, as I said above, many physicians think TSS has gone away since there is not much media attention. If I could do only one thing, I would make sure everyone in the world knows what TSS is… it is why folks die from *Staphylococcus aureus* and Group A streptococci.

Some persons have asked me what the true incidence of TSS is. Well, that all depends. As I have consistently said: Persons who die of *Staphylococcus aureus* and Group A streptococci die of pyrogenic toxin superantigens. That is a lot of persons. In 2007, the CDC stated that *Staphylococcus aureus* is the most significant cause of serious infections and infectious diseases deaths in the United States.[9] I have already mentioned that there are over five hundred thousand cases of surgical site infections, seventy thousand cases of staphylococcal pneumonia with a 60 percent fatality rate, forty thousand cases of sepsis and infective endocarditis with 50 percent fatalities. This does not count the large numbers of bone infections, where *Staphylococcus aureus* causes 90 percent, and the incredible numbers of infections in diabetic patients and those with atopic dermatitis. And what about all of those we do not recognize as caused by *Staphylococcus aureus*? However, if we want to speak about diseases, both staphylococcal and Group A streptococcal, that we would call TSS, probable TSS, or likely to be TSS (as in toxin-mediated disease), I have made the calculation that this number should be about one in five thousand per year. This translates into sixty-four thousand cases of staphylococcal and streptococcal TSS each year in the United States. If you figure we live on average eighty-five years, this means you have approximately a one in fifty chance of having TSS. This is why I say you know one or more persons who have had these diseases. This number is also not likely to be far off. The number is based on the percentage of people with protective antibodies, the age of individuals, the colonization frequency with the microbes, and the ability of the microbes to produce enough pyrogenic toxin superantigens to cross the skin or mucous membrane barriers and cause TSS symptoms. This is a lot of people each year.

I want to return briefly to menstrual, vaginal staphylococcal TSS since this is where we started. At its peak, the incidence was one woman in ten thousand developing menstrual TSS. This is exactly the expected rate based on my calculations. What is the incidence today you might ask? The incidence is about one in one hundred thousand, or ten-fold less. Remember, there are all kinds of TSS, for example there are an estimated thirty-five thousand cases of streptococcal TSS each year. The most common type of staphylococcal TSS is likely to be post-influenza TSS, and there may be thousands of cases—just not recognized for what they are.

What about the CDC? Their name is now the Centers for Disease Control and Prevention. They have thus picked up extra work. My experience in working with the CDC recently has been better. They have improved remarkably in some cases. Time will tell when new diseases arise, how well the CDC responds. I think it is telling that the CDC appears to be marginalized in the United States handling of COVID-19. I agree with this decision since their arrogance delayed deployment of a valuable diagnostic kit to detect infection for four to six weeks. It is always important to emphasize that they work for you, not the other way around. I am completely sure that they are underfunded!

What about the NIH? As I have said above, the grant review panels, called Study Sections, are housed in the Center for Scientific Review. For the most part in my area, they are bad! I have contacted the head of the Center for Scientific Review many times, so they know my thoughts. The problems are many in grant reviews. Here are a few.

Some grant review administrators have cheated, and some likely do now. They have told grant review Study Section members who to vote for and who to give great scores to so they will be funded. This is usually their friends. This can be subtle or not so subtle as one grant review administrator tried to do to me.

Some Study Section members are part of a "club" having trained with a certain now deceased professor. They have had continuous meetings, where they remind members of the club to be sure to fund their group and then fund others only if there is money left over.

Congress should examine the Study Sections carefully, not just assuming they function effectively. I have given many examples where they do not work correctly. At the NIH, the Study Sections are the only part of the NIH that are not under the control of the Office of Research Integrity. Who is more important at the NIH than Study Sections to be under this control? Scientists are people too, and they don't necessarily behave honestly. When I was chair of a Study Section at the NIH, we let some reviewers go for lack of integrity.

Most importantly for you, I think the composition of the Study Sections must change, and the things that reviewers think important must align with human health. Too many grants are funded with only lip service to human health. You should benefit from funded grants, period! If you don't, then let's move on to some other grants that are more important.

My thoughts here may require that Study Section composition be changed a lot. It is likely that the NIH will need to hire a group of experts and pay them well to do this review job. Take the reviews out of the hands of those folks with vested interest to keep their areas and universities important, when in fact they may not be important. It is important to give more than lip service to human health. I have had so many folks tell me that I have recently had trouble gaining renewal funding because I am doing applied research for human health instead of basic research into how bacteria function.

Sorry, I am perfectly able to do both applied and basic at the same time. I have now often resorted to saying: "Isn't it surprising that I have managed to publish over 450 manuscripts without your help?"

My last rant here follows. I do this sometimes to teach students, and they tell me they love it so here goes.

About fifteen years ago, I wrote a grant application in response to an NIH "Request for Applications" to study defense against bioterrorism. The application took me a year to write and was 1,475 single-spaced, 11-point font, 0.5-inch margin pages. This amount is roughly ten times the length of this book. I had to send in six paper copies to the NIH. The paper copies stood four feet tall when stacked together.

I know what happened in the grant review because, as I said, leaks happen in the Federal Government. I was told the grant application received a highly favorable review. The NIH, however, did not want to fund this, as I was not an MD or MD/PhD. Thus, they chose a second, impressively negative group of reviewers and had the application re-reviewed. One year of my life went out the window, as the grant application was not funded. What idiocy!

With TSS, I was in at the start. It looks like I am also in at the end. I have mentioned many things that have been done and many that remain to be done, related to all kinds of new diseases. I have little hope that these will be investigated. I no longer think the NIH has the will to pursue these important areas.

I am sure they lack the will, as all of my recent grant applications have been turned down. PS: To those of you with memory losses due to TSS, it will come back in a year and a half; PPS: To those of you with new diseases, expect us never to understand how they occur. My last statement: Seven years ago, I applied for a grant to study a compound that was safe for application to mucosal surfaces like nose, throat, and vagina. This compound kills 100 percent of enveloped viruses on contact. Some enveloped viruses are HIV, HSV, influenza, mumps, yellow fever virus, Ebola... and of course coronavirus. This molecule could have gone through all needed testing by now and be available for use in high-risk populations for COVID-19 in nursing homes, hospitals, home care, and cruise ships. The grant review panel said: "This is the grant application most likely to be successful. However, it is not as innovative as this other one, so we will not fund the Schlievert grant." The "other" one was made up, faked data! Need I say more?

Thank you for reading this book. Please share the information
so the world will know. Best to you!

Pat

Short Biography:

Dr. Patrick M. Schlievert received his bachelor's (geology/general science) and PhD (microbiology studying the first defensin) degrees from the University of Iowa. He was a postdoctoral associate at the University of Minnesota from 1976-1979, studying streptococcal scarlet fever toxins as causes of scarlet fever and related more serious illnesses. In 1979, Dr. Schlievert accepted a faculty position at UCLA in the Microbiology and Immunology Department, where he discovered toxic shock syndrome (TSS) toxin-1, the principle cause of TSS, and demonstrated the main reason why tampons are associated with TSS. Dr. Schlievert returned to the University of Minnesota as a faculty member in the Microbiology Department, where he worked his way through the ranks to full professor in 1990. From 2011 to 2019, he was Chair of Microbiology and Immunology and Professor of Internal Medicine at the University of Iowa. He is currently a Professor of Microbiology and Immunology and Internal Medicine. Dr. Schlievert and his clinical colleagues have described many new toxin-associated human illnesses including streptococcal TSS (the flesh-eating streptococcal disease) in 1987. His major current interests continue in description of new diseases, drug discovery, and vaccine development. Dr. Schlievert has published over 450 scientific manuscripts. While at the University of Minnesota, he taught one-third of all medical students ever trained at the university, and he received the university's highest education honor for teaching microbiology and immunology. In 2016, Dr. Schlievert was named the American Society for Microbiology Educator of the Year. He was also a member of the Academic Health Center Academy of Excellence in Medical Research at the University of Minnesota.

Dr. Patrick M. Schlievert

Selected References

1 Spaulding AR, Salgado-Pabón W, Kohler PL, Horswill AR, Leung DY, Schlievert PM. Staphylococcal and streptococcal superantigen exotoxins. Clin Microbiol Rev 2013;26:422-47.

2 Dinges MM, Orwin PM, Schlievert PM. Exotoxins of *Staphylococcus aureus*. Clin Microbiol Rev 2000;13:16-34, table of contents.

3 McCormick JK, Yarwood JM, Schlievert PM. Toxic shock syndrome and bacterial superantigens: an update. Annu Rev Microbiol 2001;55:77-104.

4 Schlievert PM, Davis CC. Device-associated menstrual toxic shock syndrome. Clin Microbiol Rev 2020;33.

5 Osterholm MT, Davis JP, Gibson RW, et al. Tri-state toxic-state syndrome study. I. Epidemiologic findings. J Infect Dis 1982;145:431-40.

6 MacDonald KL, Osterholm MT, Hedberg CW, et al. Toxic shock syndrome. A newly recognized complication of influenza and influenzalike illness. JAMA 1987;257:1053-8.

7 Schrock CG. Disease alert. Jama 1980;243:1231.

8 Schlievert PM, Shands KN, Dan BB, Schmid GP, Nishimura RD. Identification and characterization of an exotoxin from *Staphylococcus aureus* associated with toxic-shock syndrome. J Infect Dis 1981;143:509-16.

9 Klevens RM, Morrison MA, Nadle J, et al. Invasive methicillin-resistant *Staphylococcus aureus* infections in the United States. JAMA 2007;298:1763-71.

10 Vergeront JM, Stolz SJ, Crass BA, Nelson DB, Davis JP, Bergdoll MS. Prevalence of serum antibody to staphylococcal enterotoxin F among Wisconsin residents: implications for toxic-shock syndrome. J Infect Dis 1983;148:692-8.

11 Schlievert PM, Chuang-Smith ON, Peterson ML, Cook LC, Dunny GM. *Enterococcus faecalis* endocarditis severity in rabbits is reduced by IgG Fabs interfering with aggregation substance. PLoS One 2010;5.

12 Salgado-Pabón W, Schlievert PM. Models matter: the search for an effective *Staphylococcus aureus* vaccine. Nat Rev Microbiol 2014;12:585-91.

13 Cone LA, Woodard DR, Schlievert PM, Tomory GS. Clinical and bacteriologic observations of a toxic shock-like syndrome due to *Streptococcus pyogenes*. N Engl J Med 1987;317:146-9.

14 Stevens DL, Tanner MH, Winship J, et al. Severe group A streptococcal infections associated with a toxic shock-like syndrome and scarlet fever toxin A. N Engl J Med 1989;321:1-7.

15 Schlievert PM, Blomster DA. Production of staphylococcal pyrogenic exotoxin type C: influence of physical and chemical factors. J Infect Dis 1983;147:236-42.

16 Todd J, Fishaut M, Kapral F, Welch T. Toxic-shock syndrome associated with phage-group-I Staphylococci. Lancet 1978;2:1116-8.

17 Assimacopoulos AP, Strandberg KL, Rotschafer JH, Schlievert PM. Extreme pyrexia and rapid death due to *Staphylococcus aureus* infection: analysis of 2 cases. Clin Infect Dis 2009;48:612-4.

18 Larkin SM, Williams DN, Osterholm MT, Tofte RW, Posalaky Z. Toxic shock syndrome: clinical, laboratory, and pathologic findings in nine fatal cases. Ann Intern Med 1982;96:858-64.

19 Morens DM, Taubenberger JK, Fauci AS. Predominant role of bacterial pneumonia as a cause of death in pandemic influenza: implications for pandemic influenza preparedness. J Infect Dis 2008;198:962-70.

20 Schlossberg D, Kandra J, Kreiser J. Possible Kawasaki disease in a 20-year-old woman. Arch Dermatol 1979;115:1435-6.

21 Aranow H, Wood WB. Staphylococcal infection simulating scarlet fever. JAMA 1942;119:1491-5.

22 Leung DY, Schlievert PM, Meissner HC. The immunopathogenesis and management of Kawasaki syndrome. Arthritis Rheum 1998;41:1538-47.

23 Leung DY, Meissner HC, Fulton DR, Murray DL, Kotzin BL, Schlievert PM. Toxic shock syndrome toxin-secreting *Staphylococcus aureus* in Kawasaki syndrome. Lancet 1993;342:1385-8.

[24] Williams M. The Velveteen Rabbit. 1922. Simon & Schuster.

[25] Schlievert PM, Bettin KM, Watson DW. Effect of antipyretics on group A streptococcal pyrogenic exotoxin fever production and ability to enhance lethal endotoxin shock. Proc Soc Exp Biol Med 1978;157:472-5.

[26] Vu BG, Stach CS, Kulhankova K, Salgado-Pabón W, Klingelhutz AJ, Schlievert PM. Chronic superantigen exposure induces systemic inflammation, elevated bloodstream endotoxin, and abnormal glucose tolerance in rabbits: possible role in diabetes. MBio 2015;6:e02554.

[27] Mueller EA, Merriman JA, Schlievert PM. Toxic shock syndrome toxin-1, not alpha-toxin, mediated Bundaberg fatalities. Microbiology 2015;161:2361-8.

[28] Bergdoll MS, Crass BA, Reiser RF, Robbins RN, Davis JP. A new staphylococcal enterotoxin, enterotoxin F, associated with toxic-shock-syndrome *Staphylococcus aureus* isolates. Lancet 1981;1:1017-21.

[29] Schlievert PM. Enhancement of host susceptibility to lethal endotoxin shock by staphylococcal pyrogenic exotoxin type C. Infect Immun 1982;36:123-8.

[30] Parsonnet J, Hansmann MA, Delaney ML, et al. Prevalence of toxic shock syndrome toxin 1-producing *Staphylococcus aureus* and the presence of antibodies to this superantigen in menstruating women. J Clin Microbiol 2005;43:4628-34.

[31] Schlievert PM. Alteration of immune function by staphylococcal pyrogenic exotoxin type C: possible role in toxic-shock syndrome. J Infect Dis 1983;147:391-8.

[32] Marrack P, Kappler J. The staphylococcal enterotoxins and their relatives. Science 1990;248:705-11.

[33] Li H, Llera A, Tsuchiya A, et al. Three-dimensional structure of the complex between a T cell receptor beta chain and the superantigen staphylococcal enterotoxin B. Immunity 1998;9:807-16.

[34] Li Y, Li H, Dimasi N, et al. Crystal structure of a superantigen bound to the high-affinity, zinc-dependent site on MHC class II. Immunity 2001;14:93-104.

[35] Leder L, Llera A, Lavoie PM, et al. A mutational analysis of the binding of staphylococcal enterotoxins B and C3 to the T cell receptor beta chain and major histocompatibility complex class II. J Exp Med 1998;187:823-33.

[36] Malchiodi EL, Eisenstein E, Fields BA, et al. Superantigen binding to a T cell receptor beta chain of known three-dimensional structure. J Exp Med 1995;182:1833-45.

[37] McCormick JK, Tripp TJ, Llera AS, et al. Functional analysis of the TCR binding domain of toxic shock syndrome toxin-1 predicts further diversity in MHC class II/superantigen/TCR ternary complexes. J Immunol 2003;171:1385-92.

[38] Fields BA, Malchiodi EL, Li H, et al. Crystal structure of a T-cell receptor beta-chain complexed with a superantigen. Nature 1996;384:188-92.

[39] Sundberg EJ, Andersen PS, Schlievert PM, Karjalainen K, Mariuzza RA. Structural, energetic, and functional analysis of a protein-protein interface at distinct stages of affinity maturation. Structure 2003;11:1151-61.

[40] Sundberg EJ, Li H, Llera AS, et al. Structures of two streptococcal superantigens bound to TCR beta chains reveal diversity in the architecture of T cell signaling complexes. Structure 2002;10:687-99.

[41] Johnson LP, Schlievert PM. Group A streptococcal phage T12 carries the structural gene for pyrogenic exotoxin type A. Mol Gen Genet 1984;194:52-6.

[42] Roetzer A, Jilma B, Eibl MM. Vaccine against toxic shock syndrome in a first-in-man clinical trial. Expert Rev Vaccines 2017;16:81-3.

[43] Shilts R. And the Band Played On: Politics, People, and the Aids Epidemic. 1987. Penguin Books.

[44] Garrett L. The Coming Plague. 1994. Penguin Books.

[45] Schlievert P, Johnson W, Galask RP. Isolation of a low-molecular-weight antibacterial system from human amniotic fluid. Infect Immun 1976;14:1156-66.

[46] Tierno PM, Hanna BA. Enzymic hydrolysis of tampon carboxymethylcellulose and toxic shock syndrome. Lancet 1983;1:1379-80.

47 Lindsay JA, Ruzin A, Ross HF, Kurepina N, Novick RP. The gene for toxic shock toxin is carried by a family of mobile pathogenicity islands in *Staphylococcus aureus*. Mol Microbiol 1998;29:527-43.

48 Friedrich EG, Jr., Siegesmund KA. Tampon-associated vaginal ulcerations. Obstet Gynecol 1980;55:149-56.

49 Yarwood JM, McCormick JK, Schlievert PM. Identification of a novel two-component regulatory system that acts in global regulation of virulence factors of *Staphylococcus aureus*. J Bacteriol 2001;183:1113-23.

50 Tierno PM, Jr., Hanna BA. Viscose rayon versus cotton tampons. J Infect Dis 1998;177:824-6.

51 Schlievert PM. Comparison of cotton and cotton/rayon tampons for effect on production of toxic shock syndrome toxin. J Infect Dis 1995;172:1112-4.

52 Parsonnet J, Modern PA, Giacobbe KD. Effect of tampon composition on production of toxic shock syndrome toxin-1 by *Staphylococcus aureus* in vitro. J Infect Dis 1996;173:98-103.

53 Fischetti VA, Chapman F, Kakani R, James J, Grun E, Zabriskie JB. Role of air in growth and production of toxic shock syndrome toxin 1 by *Staphylococcus aureus* in experimental cotton and rayon tampons. Rev Infect Dis 1989;11 Suppl 1:S176-81.

54 Kreiswirth BN, Schlievert PM, Novick RP. Evaluation of coagulase-negative staphylococci for ability to produce toxic shock syndrome toxin 1. J Clin Microbiol 1987;25:2028-9.

55 Blomster-Hautamaa DA, Kreiswirth BN, Kornblum JS, Novick RP, Schlievert PM. The nucleotide and partial amino acid sequence of toxic shock syndrome toxin-1. J Biol Chem 1986;261:15783-6.

56 Blomster-Hautamaa DA, Novick RP, Schlievert PM. Localization of biologic functions of toxic shock syndrome toxin-1 by use of monoclonal antibodies and cyanogen bromide-generated toxin fragments. J Immunol 1986;137:3572-6.

57 Bergdoll MSaS, P.M. Toxic-shock syndrome toxin. Lancet 1984;ii:691.

58 Schlievert PM, Case LC, Nemeth KA, et al. Alpha and beta chains of hemoglobin inhibit production of *Staphylococcus aureus* exotoxins. Biochemistry 2007;46:14349-58.

59 Schlievert PM, Nemeth KA, Davis CC, Peterson ML, Jones BE. *Staphylococcus aureus* exotoxins are present in vivo in tampons. Clin Vaccine Immunol 2010;17:722-7.

60 Cockerill FR, 3rd, MacDonald KL, Thompson RL, et al. An outbreak of invasive group A streptococcal disease associated with high carriage rates of the invasive clone among school-aged children. JAMA 1997;277:38-43.

61 Goshorn SC, Bohach GA, Schlievert PM. Cloning and characterization of the gene, speC, for pyrogenic exotoxin type C from *Streptococcus pyogenes*. Mol Gen Genet 1988;212:66-70.

62 Kaul R, McGeer A, Norrby-Teglund A, et al. Intravenous immunoglobulin therapy for streptococcal toxic shock syndrome—a comparative observational study. The Canadian Streptococcal Study Group. Clin Infect Dis 1999;28:800-7.

63 Bernstein JM, Ballow M, Schlievert PM, Rich G, Allen C, Dryja D. A superantigen hypothesis for the pathogenesis of chronic hyperplastic sinusitis with massive nasal polyposis. Am J Rhinol 2003;17:321-6.

64 Jackow CM, Cather JC, Hearne V, Asano AT, Musser JM, Duvic M. Association of erythrodermic cutaneous T-cell lymphoma, superantigen-positive *Staphylococcus aureus*, and oligoclonal T-cell receptor V beta gene expansion. Blood 1997;89:32-40.

65 Spaulding AR, Salgado-Pabón W, Merriman JA, et al. Vaccination Against *Staphylococcus aureus* Pneumonia. J Infect Dis 2014;209:1955-62.

66 Kravitz GR, Dries DJ, Peterson ML, Schlievert PM. Purpura fulminans due to *Staphylococcus aureus*. Clin Infect Dis 2005;40:941-7.